SCIENCE OVER STIGMA

Education and Advocacy for Mental Health

SCIENCE OVER STIGMA

Education and Advocacy for Mental Health

Daniel B. Morehead, M.D.

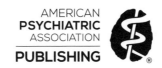

AMERICAN
PSYCHIATRIC
ASSOCIATION
PUBLISHING ®

If you wish to buy 50 or more copies of the same title, please go to www.appi.org/specialdiscounts for more information.

Copyright © 2021 American Psychiatric Association Publishing
ALL RIGHTS RESERVED
First Edition
Manufactured in the United States of America on acid-free paper
25 24 23 22 21   5 4 3 2 1
American Psychiatric Association Publishing
800 Maine Avenue SW
Suite 900
Washington, DC 20024-2812
www.appi.org

Library of Congress Cataloging-in-Publication Data
Names: Morehead, Daniel B., author. | American Psychiatric Association Publishing, issuing body.
Title: Science over stigma : education and advocacy for mental health / Daniel B. Morehead.
Description: First edition. | Washington, DC : American Psychiatric Association Publishing, [2021] | Includes bibliographical references and index.
Identifiers: LCCN 2021003320 (print) | LCCN 2021003321 (ebook) | ISBN 9781615373079 (paperback ; alk. paper) | ISBN 9781615373819 (ebook)
Subjects: MESH: Mental Disorders | Mental Health Services | Social Stigma | Patient Advocacy
Classification: LCC RC454 (print) | LCC RC454 (ebook) | NLM WM 140 | DDC 616.89—dc23
LC record available at https://lccn.loc.gov/2021003320
LC ebook record available at https://lccn.loc.gov/2021003321

British Library Cataloguing in Publication Data
A CIP record is available from the British Library.

Contents

About the Author

Daniel B. Morehead, M.D., is a psychiatrist in private practice in Austin, Texas, and Boston, Massachusetts. He speaks regularly for mental health advocacy and is clinical assistant professor of psychiatry at Tufts University Medical Center. He is also former assistant residency director at the Menninger Clinic, where he received the William C. Menninger Teaching Award. He is board certified in General Psychiatry and Neuropsychiatry and maintains interests in brain science, psychotherapy, and spirituality.

Acknowledgments

This book began many years ago with a talk for a local faith community (requested by my wife, who happened to be a minister there). Four people attended. The next occasion occurred at a community mental health conference, where organizers were surprised to receive a capacity crowd of 800 attendees. And so I would first like to thank Rev. Carol Morehead and Fonda Latham, M.S.W., the accomplished leaders who initiated my participation in their advocacy programs. In a similar way, I am grateful to Karen Ranus of NAMI, Kay Warren of Saddleback Church, Barbara Johnson, John McFarland, J.D., Carol and Don Hollins, Douglas Brown, Dan Chun, M.Div., Laura Roberts M.D., and many others for taking a chance on my ability to advocate and giving me opportunities to do so.

The generous people who reviewed the manuscript for this book surely deserve some special (yet to be specified) reward: JT. Kittridge, Charles Morehead, David Morehead, M.D., Marcia Morehead, M.S.W., Andy Montgomery, Manley Clodfelter, M.D., Kim Paffenroth, Ph.D., Don Stephenson, Lisa Madsen, M.D., Allan Cole, Ph.D., Steve Sonnenberg, M.D., and Paul Summergrad, M.D. The later two, along with Glen Gabbard, M.D., have offered vital mentoring and encouragement along the way, for which I will always be grateful. Doug Beach of NAMI has been especially energetic in his support and encouragement, and for me represents the tireless efforts of so many advocates over so many years, efforts that continue to bear fruit.

All advocacy springs from the work of those who have gone before us: Those who have experienced mental illness, their families, advocates, and helpers and treaters of all kinds (from caretakers to doctors and nurses). All of us who care about mental health owe them a profound debt. Personally, I will be forever indebted to my own patients, who have been the most patient and humble of teachers. Most of all, I want to acknowledge the scientists whose work provides the foundation for this book. Nothing in the text that follows is truly original; everything is drawn from the patient and painstaking work of numberless researchers in the fields of psychiatry, medicine, psychology, sociology, and spirituality. A few of them are famous, but we owe just as much to those whose names we will never know. All of them have devoted numberless hours and care to the vast edifice of research and clinical experience that now rises before us in the field of mental health. This achievement—truly scientific, humane understanding and treatment of mental illness—will fill us with joy and optimism, if only we have the eyes to see it.

Daniel B. Morehead, M.D.

Disclosure of Competing Interests

Dr. Morehead has indicated that he has no financial interests or other affiliations that represent or could appear to represent a competing interest with his contributions to this book.

Foreword

In 1979, a small but determined group of mothers desperate to help their children convened around a kitchen table in Madison, Wisconsin. Each parent had a child living with a mental illness and little support at the time to help their children, and themselves, so they turned to one another for comfort.

What they found was much more.

The dedicated group of parents exchanged what they had learned about mental illness, listened to one another as they talked through the painful challenges they faced, and planted seeds of a community rooted in their shared experiences. They eventually came to understand that it's okay to not be okay—and that what they were going through was more normal than they previously believed.

Realizing others could benefit from a similar peer model, the families transformed this inaugural kitchen table convening into what is now known as NAMI, the National Alliance on Mental Illness. NAMI is now a far-reaching network of more than 600 local affiliates. Along the way, NAMI created a roadmap to raising awareness about mental illness that focuses on education, community, and empathy.

We continue to use this model at NAMI. As CEO, I've seen firsthand how far the medical and advocacy communities have come in raising awareness about mental illness. But the business of changing hearts and minds on this issue is hard work, and there is still much to be done to overcome the stigma, shame, and discrimination that prevents people from accepting that mental illness is real and treatable.

That's why I could not be more grateful for Dr. Dan Morehead's book, and especially at this moment in history. The COVID-19 pandemic and the impacts of physical distancing and quarantining—science-based measures for preventing infection—have likewise taken a toll on the mental health community and people's ability to access and lean on their support systems for help. As mental health providers see an unprecedented spike in people seeking mental health care and as uncertainty remains about the long-lasting effects of the public health crisis, now more than ever we must understand how to educate, build community, and promote empathy about mental illness even as we live in isolation.

With *Science Over Stigma: Education and Advocacy for Mental Illness*, Dr. Morehead's work at the intersection of brain science, psychotherapy, and spirituality is on full display and comes together in a book perfectly designed to help health professionals educate and advocate while also being accessible to all readers. This is so very important, as we can all stand to benefit from increasing our understanding of mental illness and its reach and impact.

Early in the book, Dr. Morehead illustrates for us how common and far-reaching mental illness is. Mental illness is so common, that whether we realize it or not, we are all impacted by it — if not directly, then through someone we love, care about, live near, or work with. Today, one in five U.S. adults experiences mental illness, with anxiety disorders, depression, and post-traumatic stress disorder being among the most common. One in 20 U.S. adults lives with serious mental illness. In fact, at least 8.4 million Americans provide care to an adult with emotional or mental illness and, on average, spend 32 hours per week providing *unpaid* care.

The individual and family impact of mental illness produces a ripple effect in our communities. More than one in three people incarcerated in state and federal prisons have been diagnosed with a mental illness, and seven out of 10 youth in the juvenile justice system have at least one mental health condition. Furthermore, more than one in five people who experience homelessness, and one in eight of all visits to emergency rooms, in the United States are related to mental health and substance use disorders.

And yet, even with such far-reaching impacts, nearly 60 percent of adults with a mental illness did not receive mental health services in the previous year.[1] So while over the past few decades there has been tremendous scientific progress, as Dr. Morehead details throughout this book, the science community cannot alone improve outcomes for people living with mental illness. Scientific advances must be supported with social progress and by overcoming the stigma associated with mental illness. With that said, perhaps the most important takeaway from this book is this: You are not alone, and suffering from mental illness is nobody's fault (see Chapter 6, "Mental Illness Is Serious," and Chapter 7, "Mental Illness Is Nobody's Fault"). We are all in this together, and we all have a responsibility to fight this fight against stigma.

---

[1]NAMI: "Mental Health Facts in America." Available at: https://www.nami.org/nami/media/nami-media/infographics/generalmhfacts.pdf.

The good news: There's strength in numbers, and together can we increase the visibility of mental illness and decrease stigma. Dr. Morehead understands that because of the nature and ubiquity of mental illness, this requires a multimodal approach that must include improved individual clinical treatment and patient care, as led by the medical community and health care providers. But overcoming stigma also requires strong community-based advocacy.

Thousands of trained NAMI volunteers host peer-led programs and support groups, which include NAMI Family-to-Family, NAMI Basics, NAMI Homefront, and NAMI Provider. These programs offer training and support to caregivers, families, military service members and veterans, and mental health professionals, because it's imperative that we all become advocates—from family members, friends, and neighbors; to doctors, health care providers, and health insurance companies; to grasstops and grassroots organizers and organizations, community leaders, judges, and legislators at all levels of government. Each of us has a role to play.

In the past few years, we've seen how well a multimodal approach to overcoming stigma works. Tremendous improvements in the availability of mental health treatment have been accompanied and enhanced by a momentous cultural breakthrough.

When Prince Harry stepped outside of royal tradition and opened up about his decades-long mental health struggle and how he dealt with it, his story made headline news.[2] The world took notice again when last summer, former First Lady Michelle Obama shared on her podcast that she was experiencing low-grade depression and how quarantining from COVID-19 and social and civil unrest had left her feeling "too low."[3]

But we can also look a little closer to home to bear witness to the sea change in attitudes toward mental illness and health, as young people across the country have been among our best teachers (see Chapter 8, "Mental Illness Is Treatable"). As Dr. Morehead points out and suggests, mental illness usually begins early in life—when people are teenagers or young adults—and that deep wisdom lies in the excruciatingly painful experiences of coming of age while suffering from mental illness. And it's true. Social media

---

[2]Rodriguez C: "Prince Harry Opens Up About His 20-Year Mental Struggle." Forbes April 18, 2017. Available at: https://www.forbes.com/sites/ceciliarodriguez/2017/04/18/prince-harry-opens-up-about-his-20-years-of-mental-struggle/?sh=45dce2f378ab.
[3]Taylor DB: Michelle Obama Says She Is Dealing With 'Low-Grade Depression.'" New York Times August 6, 2020; updated August 18, 2020. Available at: https://www.nytimes.com/2020/08/06/us/michelle-obama-depression.html.

provides an accessible and often free platform to educate, build community, and express empathy. Young people regularly turn to social media to express themselves, and they have not precluded talking openly about their own mental health struggles, sharing their therapist's advice, or expressing when they too are suffering through acute symptoms associated with mental illness on these platforms. As a result, these candid exchanges are lifesaving.

There is a valuable lesson to be learned from this transformative cultural shift, and that is, we must all be available to give one another grace: the grace to acknowledge that we or someone we love or care about is suffering from a mental illness; the grace to give ourselves an opportunity to learn more about mental health and the impact of mental illness; and the grace to build support systems and get the help we need and deserve.

It has not been easy to shift an entire culture on this issue. This cultural progress did not come without improved early-intervention methods, people increasingly having frank conversations with their health care providers about their mental health as a matter of course, and providers incorporating treatment into their patients' health care plans.

And that speaks to what this book does best, which is to reaffirm that combating mental illness is a systemwide effort. And if there's one thing I know for sure is that it will take all of us pulling the levers of science, policy, medicine, and culture to pierce the veil of stigma, shame, and discrimination that surrounds mental illness.

Daniel H. Gillison Jr.
Chief Executive Officer, NAMI
January 2021

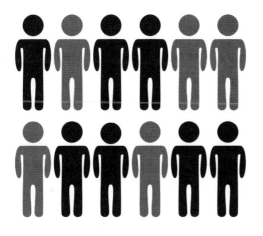

Introduction

Education and Advocacy for Mental Illness: Why Bother?

Our country is of two minds about mental illness. On the one hand, people of the United States overwhelmingly endorse the idea that mental illness is real medical illness. A near-unanimous public majority maintains that mental illness is both real (97%) and treatable (86%–95%) (American Psychological Association 2019; Universal Health Services 2019). One recent poll showed that 87% assert that mental health disorders are "nothing to be ashamed of" (American Psychological Association 2019). And a surprising 71%–89% classify mental and physical health as equally important (Research American 2006; Universal Health Services 2019).

People agree that mental illness is real. On the other hand, people act as if mental illness is not real. If public opinion has steadily shifted toward a recognition of psychiatric illness, public behavior has not. Less than half of people with diagnosable mental illness get treatment in any given year (Substance Abuse and Mental Health Services Administration 2018), and this number has changed little in nearly two decades (Wang et al. 2005). Of those who do get treatment, only about half adhere to it (Sajatovic et al. 2010). Thus, the vast majority of people with mental illness do not accept treatment for it, and do not fully accept the medical necessity of such treatment.

This radical inconsistency of thought and action should not surprise any mental health professional. The contradiction between belief and behavior lay at the root of Freud's insights about the unconscious, and continued in the "split brain" experiments of Gazzaniga and Sperry that heralded the beginning of modern neuropsychology. It is part of the daily fare of mental health practitioners. Put simply, it is possible to know one thing and do another. Our brain systems for conscious understanding seem to operate along different pathways from those for feeling and motivation. When these contradictions become unbearable, we seek mental health treatment or other forms of growth and healing. Even so, self-contradictory behaviors are a fixture of human nature and can become embarrassingly obvious in both individual and community life. To say one thing and do another is simply a part of the human condition.

Although I cannot prove it, I see the opposite contradiction in the current culture of mental health professionals. On the one hand, we seem to act every bit as if mental illness is real medical illness. Everywhere I look, I see colleagues going about their business in a straightforward, rational, scientifically grounded manner. I see all sorts of health professionals, from primary care physicians to social workers, treating mental health conditions as medical illnesses with medical treatments. Every day, I see psychotherapists recommending medications and pharmacotherapists recommending talk therapy. Although our field is fraught with challenges, I do not generally see massive overdiagnosis, overmedication, or overreliance on just one form of treatment. Nor do I see any crisis of confidence that prevents us from diagnosing and treating mental illnesses in a vigorous manner. Instead, I see a steadily maturing field of mostly well-trained, thoughtful clinicians who go about their business according to appropriate professional and scientific standards.

On the other hand, while mental health professionals act as if mental illness is treatable and real, we regularly speak as if it is not. Of course, in an implicit sense, almost all clinicians "know" that mental illness is real and treatable. It is in our bones and in our guts, a reality that is usually too obvious for words. Most of us do not spend time debating the nature of mental illness any more than surgeons spend time debating the reality or definition of medical illness. We sense clearly enough that it is real and that we need to get on with treating it.

Even so, when we begin to talk explicitly about mental illness, our professional culture begins to sound radically uncertain. We rarely articulate the confidence we enact in clinical practice. For instance, it is commonplace to assert that we cannot generally define mental illness. Some academic experts have even asserted that we should give up trying (Phillips et al. 2012). It is just as common to assert that we do not know the neurobiology of our most important mental illnesses. We do not know the central pathophysiology of major depression, or the neurobiological cause of schizophrenia, or why some people get PTSD and others do not. So (it is said) we cannot even define what we are treating, philosophically or medically. In similar fashion, debates about the reality of various mental illnesses regularly resurface, even among medical professionals (Pies 2015). *The New England Journal of Medicine*, for instance, occasionally features articles debating whether addiction is a mental illness or simply a learned behavior (Lewis 2018; Volkow et al. 2016). Meanwhile, the British Psychological Society's report on schizophrenia allowed that psychotic symptoms could amount to social deviance or simple eccentricities (Cooke 2014; Frances 2013). And, of course, there is the long-running debate over the nature and legitimacy of DSM, along with regular criticisms that psychiatry is vastly overdiagnosing and overmedicating our population (see Chapter 4).

Such literary conversations stimulate those within our field but confuse those outside it. We should not be surprised, therefore, that skepticism about psychiatry is considered sophisticated among educated Americans. Publications such as *The Atlantic*, *The New York Times*, and *The New Yorker* contain periodic features with titles like "Mental Illness Is All in Your Brain—or Is It?" (Szalai 2019) and "Psychiatry's Incurable Hubris" (Greenberg 2019). Historians continue to document the failures of psychiatry, characterizing it as frequently misguided, overconfident, and reductionistic (Harrington 2019). And there are a host of popular books that question the entire mental health enterprise, from DSM to clinical diagnosis to treatment (see Chapter 4).

Full-scale attacks on psychiatry are commonplace from both within and without, yet strangely enough, few mental health professionals think of defending it so vigorously. We rarely see anyone explaining the entire edifice of mental health diagnosis and treatment, much less defending it. I suspect this is because mental health clinicians and researchers sense that the scientific debate ended years ago. Scientific research has obviated the traditional critiques of our field, which are mostly irrelevant to both practice and research. Most of the questions that do remain relevant (such as areas of overdiagnosis or overmedication) are peripheral and not central to our craft. That is, they are questions of degree (how much to diagnose and treat) and not kind (whether to diagnose and treat at all). Most clinicians do not think of defending the legitimacy of mental illness and its treatment any more than surgeons think of defending the existence of surgery. For surgeons, the relevant question is when to utilize surgery, not whether surgery should be used at all. In the same way, clinicians think actively about when to diagnose and apply treatments for mental illness and are usually quite skillful in helping patients understand their plight. But few of us think about mental health practice in a general way or feel compelled to explain the generalities to patients and their families.

What results is a strange dichotomy in our culture: Clinicians treat mental illness as real but do not sound as if they know it is real. The public, on the other hand, says that mental illness is real but acts as if it is not. To be a bit more precise: The public acts confused about the nature of mental health, as well it should be, judging from public discussions of the subject. On the one hand, people rightfully accept the pronouncements of medical authorities, government agencies (such as the National Institute for Mental Health [NIMH]), and nonprofit groups (such as the National Alliance on Mental Illness [NAMI]) that mental illness is both real and treatable. On the other hand, people live with the uneasy sense that something is deeply wrong with mental health treatment, a sense fed by uncontradicted critiques of psychiatry. It is as if people viscerally know something is rotten in mental health and cannot stop searching for it. People suspect that there must be some source of corruption and mismanagement, even if they are not really sure whether there is widespread corruption and mismanagement. And people feel that psychiatry must have a shaky or nonexistent scientific basis, even as the public "oohs and aahs" over the latest neuroscience research. The public rarely hears a full explanation of our mental health practices and rarely hears about the overwhelming scientific evidence that supports such practices. And so, most people affirm the goodness of psychiatric treatment while strenuously avoiding it.

The signs of public ambivalence are not especially hard to notice: Acceptance of mental health diagnosis and treatment is growing, while at the same time rates of treatment do not increase. Understanding of mental illness is growing, yet stigma continues (Livingston and Boyd 2010; Parcesepe and Cabassa 2013). Governments and insurers now accept that mental health should be addressed as other medical problems, yet mental health treatment is handled in a drastically different fashion by both. We discriminate against mental disorders at the same time we declare such discrimination illegal. Our own patients go to great lengths to get treatment yet still feel "weak" for seeking it and ashamed of receiving it. They doubt the reality of their illnesses and the legitimacy of their treatments, regularly going on and off medications, cycling in and out of treatment. Patients, like the rest of the public, know that mental illness is real but feel as if it is not. They see the necessity of psychiatric treatment but feel that it is self-indulgent.

The national tension about mental health is not dramatic, but the results are disastrous. The ambivalence that we Americans have toward medical treatment of mental illness costs thousands of lives every year and incalculable levels of human suffering. While we accept mental illness in general, we reject those who carry it and socially distance ourselves from them (De Pinto and Backus 2019; Parcesepe and Cabassa 2013). While greater numbers of people access mental health care, deaths from substance use and suicide rise dramatically (Woolf and Schoomaker 2019). By law, insurance companies must cover mental illnesses as they do other medical problems, yet in practice this does not occur (Appelbaum and Parks 2020). Psychiatric treatment is grossly underfunded and overcontrolled by insurers and governments. For years, everyone has agreed that people with severe mental illness should receive the highest levels of treatment and social support. Yet treatment of severe mental illness in this country constitutes a scandal and a human rights disaster. Everyone knows that individuals with severe mental illness are more likely to be jailed than treated (Torrey et al. 2010). Everyone knows that treatment funding is preposterously low for those with serious illness, and yet the situation remains unaltered.

If we fully believed in the medical realities of mental illness, such events would not be tolerated. Imagine, for instance, that severe forms of cancer received no more treatment and research funding than mild forms. Imagine patients with metastatic cancer languishing in the streets because of utterly inadequate social and medical support. Imagine that all forms of treatment for *diabetes* were underfunded except for outpatient appointments and medications, leaving those with ketoacidosis, hyperglycemic crisis, and osteomyelitis to fend for themselves as outpatients. What if people with medical illness and *delirium* were regularly jailed with minimal medical care due to being combative or socially disruptive? It is difficult to imagine, because such actions violate common sense and simple humanity.

This ambivalence is costing patients dearly, and we who are mental health professionals cannot simply wait for the situation to improve. Due to the COVID-19 pandemic, the long-term situation is far more likely to worsen than improve (Vindegaard and Benros 2020). The plight of our patients is already urgent. Therefore, the plight of our profession is urgent. It is time for the second-class status of psychiatry and other mental health care to come to an end. It is time for our national ambivalence to end. It is time for half measures in the treatment of mental illness to come to an end. And it is time for us to end it. We as medical and mental health providers have the authority, the experience, and the understanding to do so. We have the instrument (science) and the means (access to our patients and communities), and the goal is well within our reach—if we have the will to take hold of it.

Who Advocates?

Honestly, I am writing a book about advocacy, yet prior to becoming involved, I would never have sought out a book or lecture on the topic. I am a psychiatrist in long-term private practice. I spend my time in individual dialogue with patients, offering psychotherapy and biological treatments to one patient at a time. Though I have spent time in academic and research settings (and continue to teach), I find my clinical work to be overwhelmingly satisfying. I do not feel a great need to be out among large groups, and I only began regular public advocacy by chance. I have since then spoken about mental illness to large and small groups of almost every description—business leaders, NAMI members, faith groups, young adults, and of course thousands of patients. Yet I never thought of myself as an advocate, or even thought that I needed to learn about advocacy.

So who advocates? Most of us have the same reflexive response: someone else. To various degrees, we all support our professional organizations, advocacy groups such as NAMI, and government agencies such as NIMH. All of these are prominent public advocates, and all of these do an excellent job. But all of them would tell us that together they are not enough. The evidence itself tells us that they are not enough. We, the community of clinicians who treat mental health disorders, are enough. We are numerous enough and influential enough to push our larger culture to a complete acceptance of the realities of mental illness and the necessities of its treatment.

Over 38,000 psychiatrists are practicing in the United States (Bishop et al. 2016). This number pales in comparison to the more than 200,000 primary care physicians (Agency for Healthcare Research and Quality 2018b) and 50,000 nurse practitioners in primary care, along with over 30,000 physician assistants (Agency for Healthcare Research and Quality 2018a). In mental health, there are more than 350,000 licensed social workers (Salsberg et al. 2017), 100,000 licensed psychologists (American Psychological Association 2014), and 250,000 mental health therapists and addiction therapists (U.S. Bureau of Labor Statistics 2019). Given these numbers, it seems safe to say that there are about a million professionals who regularly treat mental illness in this country, not including nurses, nursing assistants, crisis line workers, and mental health aides and technicians. There are too many to count, and more than enough to form a critical mass for the cultural change we need.

All of these million or so people advocate. Everyone reading this book is an advocate. Everyone who explains mental illness to a client or patient or friend advocates. Everyone who recommends a treatment for mental illness advocates. Everyone who supports family members with mental illness advocates. When we offer information to trainees, support personnel, and fellow clinicians, we advocate. When we talk to a friend about depression or a family member about alcoholism, we advocate. Most of us do not think of ourselves as advocates because we engage only in grassroots, person-to-person advocacy. We advocate unofficially and unconsciously, but this is the most important kind of advocacy. When someone we know and trust tells us about mental illness, we are inclined to listen.

And all of us together have been powerful advocates. In truth, the last couple of generations have seen astounding improvements in our cultural understanding and response to mental illness. Put another way, there has been more progress in understanding and helping those with mental illness in the last 70 years than in all eras of previous human history combined. Every advocate and every mental health professional should take justifiable pride in this fact, and every one of us should feel grateful for the generations of advocates and educators who came before us. Psychiatrists, psychologists, social workers, physicians of other medical specialties, researchers, members of NAMI, families, and people with mental illness have all contributed mightily to this cause. The medical and social treatment of those with mental illness is unrecognizable compared with treatment of the mid-twentieth century: We now have scientifically validated treatments of all major forms of mental illness. We have widely shared standards for diagnosing mental illness. Mental health care is accepted and practiced as an integral part of medical care. At least in principle, we have agreement by the government and insurers that mental illness is true medical illness. Parity between mental and medical illness is now a matter of law. The public, researchers, and medical professionals agree that mental illness is biologically and medically real. Mental illness is no longer a taboo topic in the popular culture, and sympathetic treatments appear regularly in film and television. Patients and families are empowered participants rather than helpless victims.

All of us should feel immensely proud of our collective efforts. From a wider historical view, the results have been spectacular. We should all feel proud, but at the same time we can all do better. All of us can do more in ways that are congenial to our individual personalities and habits. All of us can be better prepared to educate, more up-to-date and confident in our knowledge base. All of us can be more attentive for opportunities to advocate outside of the clinic, and braver in responding to them. All of us can be more clear, powerful, and on point in the way we present the information. All of us have community connections among extended family, groups of friends, faith communities, book clubs, volunteer organizations, sports organizations, and internet chat boards. And all of us can wield greater influence on behalf of those countless millions who face mental illness. I hope that this book will be one of many tools to help us do all of these things.

How Do We Begin?

All mental health clinicians know the following from experience: If we want to help others heal, we need to pursue healing in ourselves. We cannot offer others what we do not have. So we need to embody the change we seek to bring about in our culture. If we intend to "heal" our national ambivalence about mental health, we need to resolve our own ambivalence first.

In one way, the information in this book—and the information that the public needs—is already part of the professional DNA of every competent mental health practitioner. We all implicitly know that mental illness is real medical illness, that it is deadly serious, that treatment is anything but hopeless. But in another way, we all have our own residual doubts and biases, hindrances that keep us from true clarity on this issue and from advocating for our field in a straightforward, unhesitating way. When we and colleagues in our field still feel ashamed about our own mental illness, when so many of us still avoid full treatment of it, when so many of us have to avoid fully disclosing our mental illness to medical employers and professional organizations, it is clear that our professional culture still embodies some of the residual ambivalence that most of us carry. So I hope that this book will provide more than a review of the information we all need for advocacy and education. I hope that the reading experience will foster a full emotional conviction to accompany our intimate knowledge of the realities of mental illness. Without such emotional clarity, we will never have the motivation or the will to do the community work we need to do.

Although personal and emotional empowerment is most important, we also need conceptual clarity to advocate more effectively. We need the right information at our fingertips, and it is often different from the information that we need to practice as mental health professionals. I have tried to summarize this information as concisely as possible. All of us "know" the basic information of mental health science contained in this book, but we all need to master this information, not through a one-time review, but through a regular process of relearning and reintegration, each time at a deeper and more thorough level. I have personally been over this material hundreds of times, and each time I review it, I experience it as new, exciting, and powerful. Each time, I learn and understand it more deeply. Each time, I experience a shock of recognition, a sense that I knew this before but did not truly know and grasp the overwhelming significance of mental health for myself and everyone else in our culture.

In brief, our task is to thoroughly integrate this information into the emotional, social, and cognitive levels of our nervous systems. I do not think this task should be daunting. On a deep and intuitive level, we understand the realities of mental illness and its treatment. We could not practice effectively if we did not. We are most of the way there. But all of us have pockets of ambivalence, based on gaps in our education, personal issues with mental illness, and, most of all, old attitudes and feelings that color our current views. And we must address these old attitudes.

More than any other group, mental health practitioners understand that the past colors our view of the present. Yet, like every other discipline, psychiatry suffers from an unconscious hangover of old attitudes and old ways of thinking. Most of us seem to fall back into these when publicly speaking of mental health, even if they influence little of what we do as practitioners. Still, they confuse us and our listeners when we attempt to engage with widespread skepticism about our craft. And so we need to name and correct them.

How Not to Advocate: Avoiding Dangerous Dichotomies of the Past

These old ways of thinking reflect unreal dichotomies, "either/or" approaches that do not honor current holistic ways of understanding our field. These black-and-white characterizations usually distort the many-shaded nature of reality and use one truth to cancel out another. The history of mental health is littered with such long-running debates as genes vs. environment, conscious vs. unconscious mental life, and the importance of behavior vs. affect vs. cognition. We have to take particular care to avoid these dichotomies when speaking publicly.

Knowing Everything vs. Not Knowing Anything

We do not know the central pathology of any of the major mental illnesses, including major depression, bipolar disorder, and schizophrenia. Internal and external critics therefore assert that mental illnesses are medically unproven and unsubstantiated. Of the medical professions, psychiatry is the only one in which not knowing everything equals not knowing anything. Yet only in psychiatry (among medical specialties) does not knowing everything equal not knowing anything. But ignorance about what precisely causes depression (for instance) does not mean that depression is not medical. For centuries, doctors knew that cancer was real medical illness, even though the cause of cancer (DNA alterations) was not fully explicated until the 1960s and 1970s. Today, doctors can treat migraine headaches without knowing the precise cause. No one doubts the medical reality of migraine headaches. Similarly, we have more than enough scientific evidence that major depression is medically real and devastating, even if we do not yet have the neuropathological holy grail for the cause of depression. We know that the major mental illnesses are all associated with structural and functional brain changes, genetic contributions, cellular and subcellular dysfunction, increased inflammation, medical comorbidities, medical disability, and substantially increased mortality (see Chapters 5 and 6). There is overwhelming evidence that mental illness is real, regardless of what we still do not know about it.

In most of our public discussions, we need to remember that public debates have very different contexts from "in-house" debates. In public, there is no context to statements such as "We still do not know exactly what happens to cause depression in the brain." Or rather, the context is the vague impression that mental health treatment is based on unscientific foundations. Those outside of our field have little sense of the flood of genetic, brain imaging, microscopic, hormonal, inflammatory, functional, and epidemiological studies on mental illness, which together paint a clear picture of mental illnesses as both biological and devastating. We as mental health professionals are not going out on a limb when we assert the realities of these illnesses and their treatments, and we do not need to hide the fact that so much remains unknown. The brain is the most complicated thing in the natural world, and knowing a lot about it (as we do) does not mean we know everything about it. We know an immense amount about mental illness, and we do not know an immense amount about mental illness. Both statements are equally true. Yet what we know is more than enough to scientifically justify the diagnosis and treatment of these disorders.

Many of us who went through medical training heard the following saying countless times: "Medicine is 80% gray and 20% black-and-white—but you had better know that black-and-white." In a general way, I suspect this applies to mental health as well. There are unambiguous truths, and we should emphasize these in public discussions. Nevertheless, much of what we "know" is gray and uncertain, and we can candidly admit this at the same time.

Biology vs. Psychology

Dualistic thinking emerges during childhood and may be a part of human nature (Bloom 2005). Human beings tend to divide biological, physical events from psychological, mental ones. So even when we as mental health professionals think and speak holistically, our audiences may hear us dualistically. When we say that mental illness is as biological as cancer or diabetes, we may be heard as being reductionists who deny mental factors in mental illness. In truth, an illness that is "more" biological is not any "less" mental. The two coexist at all times and are not in competition. We can be firm about the fundamental biological dysfunction at the root of mental illness while being just as clear about the reality of psychological dysfunction in the pathophysiology and treatment of mental illness. Psychological and social realities are also real; they simply exist at a higher level of complexity than more simple biological events (Kendler 2005).

Medication vs. Psychotherapy

Psychiatry and psychology have a long history of divisions between psychologically oriented clinicians and researchers on the one hand and biologically oriented ones on the other. On one side, many pharmacologists of past generations once dismissed psychotherapy as unscientific psychobabble. On the other, many psychotherapists viewed medications as mind-numbing drugs that could never address the roots of mental illness. Many commentators continue to describe the mental health field in this way, so we as advocates need to go out of our way to dispel this view (Carlat 2010; Luhrmann 2001). Thanks to extensive scientific research, the days of such divisions are over. Psychotherapy has biological effects (Barsaglini et al. 2014), and biological treatments usually complement psychological ones. We can therefore be utterly clear about the real and effective nature of psychological and social treatments, which likewise are not less biological than medicines and neural stimulation therapies.

Psychiatry vs. Other Medical Specialties

There is a subtle but pervasive understanding, even among physicians, that psychiatry lags behind other medical specialties. Psychiatry has long been seen as less scientific, more subjective, and simply less effective than other established specialties, like oncology and ophthalmology. A common knee-jerk reaction is to view psychiatry as a second-class specialty in comparison to others. This impression, however, is superficial and outdated. Psychiatry now rests on an immensely sophisticated and rapidly deepening foundation of neuroscience. Research shows that our treatments compare well to those of other common and chronic medical conditions (Leucht et al. 2012). Yet critics routinely assume that any doubts or inconclusive data about mental health care delegitimize the entire undertaking. Why, for instance, can one negative review of antidepressant medications create a widespread sense of crisis, after decades and hundreds of studies on antidepressants (Fountoulakis et al. 2013; McAllister-Williams 2008)? And why does the same occur in regard to stimulant medications for ADHD, when studies show a high level of effectiveness for these medications (Banaschewski et al. 2016)? Studies of psychiatric medications are performed according to the same scientific standards as those for other types of medications, but the hand-wringing begins immediately when these studies are challenged, as if we share this secret conviction that our treatments are unreal and ineffective. Even if some of our treatments ultimately prove to be inadequate or misguided, this would not separate psychiatry from any other medical specialty, including oncology and gynecology (Prasad et al. 2013).

A related issue concerns attitudes about systems of psychiatric diagnosis such as DSM. Psychiatrists and other professionals have long maintained that we do not know how to precisely define or delineate mental illness. Internal and external critics of psychiatry tend to take this as *ipso facto* proof that mental illnesses are unreal, or at most the cultural creations of psychiatrists (via DSM). In fact, many philosophers of medicine also hold that we cannot precisely define and delineate medical illness (Stein 2008). Yet no one concludes that medical illnesses do not exist or that they constitute a fraud on the part of doctors. No one really believes that our difficulties defining the precise boundaries of medical illness are going to invalidate the realities of severe medical illness. However, that is precisely the conclusion that many outsiders draw about mental illnesses.

Although illnesses like chronic fatigue and fibromyalgia remain difficult to define or classify, no one attacks the credibility of rheumatology in the same way that psychiatry comes under fire for entertaining even the possibility that complicated grief or behavioral addictions might constitute mental disorders. The example of ADHD, a well-established disorder, is especially interesting. Studies have shown that ADHD is more heritable than type II diabetes, heart disease, or breast cancer and responds better to treatment than most mental and general medical illnesses (Banaschewski et al. 2016; Brikell et al. 2015), yet it remains a favorite of critics, who have by and large convinced the public that mental health professionals are creating a nation of speed addicts by treating this serious disorder. Certainly, we should regularly reevaluate the widespread diagnosis and treatment of children with putative ADHD, as well as the risks of stimulants, but areas of overdiagnosis and overtreatment do not invalidate the existence of this biological disorder, which rests on scientific data.

Mental health care will continue to grow and change over time. Treatments and diagnostic instruments we use today will become obsolete. We need both internal and external critics to help us reform and refine our practices. But when deep questions about mental health care arise, we should be wary of concluding that all mental health diagnosis and treatment is flawed. Instead, we should insist on the same standards of legitimacy for psychiatry that we do for other medical specialties.

Mild vs. Severe Mental Illness

A large portion of the public has the impression that "mental illnesses" or "biologically based mental illnesses" refer to illnesses such as schizophrenia or bipolar disorder, but not to "milder" forms such as depression or anxiety. For instance, a national poll showed that over half of people believe depression can be caused by personal weakness or failing, at the same time that 73% affirm "mental illnesses should be treated no differently from physical ones" (Kaiser Permanente 2017). While it is intuitively easier to believe that disorders like schizophrenia are the result of biological brain dysfunction, the view that various forms of depression and anxiety are not biologically based is a pernicious misunderstanding. It widens the gulf between so-called "normal" people with milder illnesses and "abnormal" people with severe ones, directly contributing to stigma.

A related issue is the tendency to unfavorably compare treatment for mild vs. severe forms of mental illness. Mental health professionals and advocates are rightly appalled at the gross underfunding of treatment for severe mental illness, but frequently contrast this with possible overtreatment of mild forms of illness in clinic settings. For instance, Allen Frances published a powerful and much-discussed piece in the *Huffington Post*, *Psychology Today*, and *Psychiatric Times* contrasting 1) "the overtreatment of the worried well" with 2) "the neglect of the really sick" by all responsible organizations (Frances 2015). Ethically, he was surely correct to juxtapose the two, but members of the public might also be forgiven for taking away the impression that those with mild to moderate mental illnesses are really the "worried well" who do not need treatment at all. Even worse, such an image puts those with severe mental illness back into their own segregated camp, unrelated to the plight of those with other forms of mental illness. In truth, everyone is in this together. Those with milder forms of depression and anxiety have mental illness, and so do those with more severe forms. All should be treated appropriately, and certainly those persons with severe illness should receive the lion's share of resources, as in every other branch of medicine.

Us vs. Them

This brings us to the most dangerous dichotomy of them all: us vs. them. The idea is that there is a different sort of person who has mental illness (such as the "schizophrenic") who is not like everybody else and who needs special pity. I feel confident from personal experience that this notion runs terrifyingly deep in our cultural attitudes, even among those with the best intentions. People have frequently attempted to encourage my advocacy with comments such as "It's so good to do something to help them" or "I feel so bad for those people." As long as those with mental illness are "them," as long as "they" are the crazy, the weird, and the helpless, attempts at advocacy will fail miserably.

Only the fundamental realization that everybody is in the same boat with regard to mental illness can change the approach to mental illness forever. The fact that around half of people will experience mental illness in their lifetime (see Chapter 3) means that having mental illness is as common as being a woman or a man. And if half the population experiences mental illness, then it is certain that everyone is affected, at least indirectly. Everyone has someone they care about who has experienced mental illness. Mental illness concerns everybody; it concerns the human condition. And once our culture has deeply integrated this one reality, a new era of mental health will finally begin.

Medically speaking, we do not culturally separate those with mild diabetes controlled by diet from those with "brittle diabetes" or advanced end-organ damage. We do not ontologically distinguish those with mild hypertension from those with malignant hypertension. Nor do we act as if treatment of people with basal cell and thyroid cancers should be in competition with treatments of metastatic cancer. Why then do we act as if severe mental illness constitutes its own unique category? I suggest that this attitude, however well intentioned, is the result of residual stigma, not progress in mental health. And it is time that those of us who advocate put an end to it.

Finally, there is one more version of the "us vs. them" dichotomy that is unique to mental health professionals. Often, in our professional roles, we forget that we too are part of the "us" affected by mental illness. The limited available evidence suggests that lifetime rates of mental illness are even higher among mental health professionals than in the general public, possibly around 70%. Similarly, mental health professionals seem more likely to experience mental illness among family members, something that prompts many of us to enter the field in the first place (see Chapter 7). Therefore, we mental health professionals *are* the ones with mental illness, at the same time that we are the ones who *treat* mental illness. We are the "them," which also means that they are the "us." On the deepest level, the line that separates us from our patients, and from the rest of the public, is an illusion. In clinical practice, we keep our personal lives separate, as we should. But as advocates, we need an implicit attitude of being one with those we address, whether they are patients, family members, or community advocates.

Thus, the important practical virtue for advocacy is humility. I hope that at least part of the time you will be advocating (and reading this book) from the perspective of someone who has mental illness, or from the perspective of a family member of someone with mental illness. Even if this is not the case, all of us who are medical and mental health professionals are deeply connected to people who have mental illness. This is a professional issue, but it is also a personal issue. And so I urge you to approach this topic from a personal perspective so that you can in turn approach people outside our field. The days of medical paternalism are over. As professionals, we are just as often suspected as trusted, and doubted as believed, by members of the public. Therefore, we need to approach community members as equals, but equals who can remind them of the scientific and personal realities of mental illness and its treatment. In other words, we professionals have just as personal an interest in mental illness as anyone else. We personally care whether mental illness is real and whether people get appropriate treatment. We are not authorities forcing our own professional interests on the public. We are members of the public who have the same interests as everyone else on these issues.

For What Do We Advocate?

The approach of this book is simple: We need to advocate by communicating the fundamental scientific basis of mental health care, a basis that most clinicians assume but do not articulate. Although we all know the following statements are true, few of us bother to regularly articulate them:

- Mental illness is common.
- Mental illness is real.
- Mental illness is serious.
- Mental illness is treatable.

These assertions would not raise an eyebrow in any mental health or even medical clinic. And members of the public recognize that these constitute the party line on mental illness (as the polls show). But members of the public seem to take these statements more as ideological beliefs than as descriptions of reality. They know they "should" believe this catechism, and they try their best to believe it. But they are not wholly convinced, and their deeper beliefs about mental illness repeatedly resurface in their behaviors. They do not realize that there is a bedrock of science supporting these assertions. They do not know that these assertions are now beyond serious scientific debate. They do not yet feel the emotional conviction that comes with deeper knowledge about the realities of mental illness and mental health. Neither do most of our intelligentsia—our journalists, historians, and cultural critics who comment on mental illness. They all need to learn, and we need to help them do so.

Rather than hearing broad generalities, members of the public need to experience a deeper, more detailed level of understanding for themselves. They need to see the science for themselves. They need to look at the numbers, the graphs, the headscan photos, and even some of the studies for themselves. Because mental health science is immensely complicated, these only amount to examples. But specific examples will carry a power far beyond that of generalities. Though most will not remember the details of such examples, they will carry away a deeper conviction that mental illness is indeed real medical illness. And perhaps for the first time, they will experience mental illness and its treatment to be grounded in reality rather than cultural consensus alone. Treatment of mental illness will then become as intuitively obvious as treatment of a broken bone or appendicitis.

Approach of the Book

"See one, do one, teach one." All of us with medical training have heard this saying, and most of us have practiced it. I often think how appalled patients would be to know that this has been a longtime refrain in our medical education system. Nevertheless, there is a great deal of wisdom in this proverbial saying. Medicine (including mental health treatment) is a practical art. It is a practical art based on science, but it is primarily about doing, not just knowing. Therefore, the best way to learn medicine is to observe it and then do it, once we know enough to understand what we are doing. I believe that advocacy is also a practical art and can best be learned in a similar fashion.

Most medical and mental health training requires spending some time in the classroom, but more time observing and practicing our art. We begin as observing students, move up to being carefully supervised interns and residents, and finally attempt to become independent practitioners and teachers of our craft. This book follows a similar principle, though in a much more modest way: The rest of this book is presented as a "see one" experience, an example of advocacy in action. Therefore I have written the bulk of each chapter as if I were addressing members of the public for the purposes of advocacy. It is meant to teach (sharpen what we know about mental illness), but even more to lay out a way of articulating and presenting the nature of mental illness and mental health treatment.

In spite of my introductory remarks, I do not believe that my colleagues need much formal training in how to speak to people, how to make an emotional connection, or how to deal with contentious issues. We as mental health professionals do these every day in clinical practice. Although admonitions such as "be concise" or "use everyday language" are correct, they do little to help us refine our ability to advocate. Personal stories and case examples are powerful tools in advocacy, but I will assume you have plenty of your own to offer. So I will offer only a smattering of these, and predominantly provide an example of advocacy for you to adapt to your own style and needs. For those seeking more specific direction, I have included a section with some practical reminders at the end of each chapter called "Advice for Advocacy." But, more importantly, I sincerely hope that you will improve upon this model as you consciously observe yourself in various forms of advocacy, and find what works for you and the specific people whom you address. All of us naturally take bits and pieces from our teachers and colleagues: sayings, attitudes, and important facts. And all of us combine and integrate them in a way that best suits our own personalities and practices.

As a "see one," the chapters that follow are "addressed" to members of the public. The illustrations and captions have been presented in the same way. That is, the language and visual aids will be suited to the general public rather than reflecting the way that mental health and medical professionals communicate with each other. As advocates, our job is not to teach mental health science, but to translate science into the vernacular and the thought world of people outside our field. Therefore, I have written the bulk of each chapter as if I were addressing members of the public for the purposes of advocacy. The introduction to each chapter is addressed directly to mental health professionals, but the remainder is "spoken" as if to the public, the objects of our advocacy. This unusual approach is meant to provide an exemplar for advocacy, a template that you can adapt to your own needs and preferences. The result, I hope, is informal and open, but not disorganized or rambling. The sequence of ideas, the vocabulary used to express them, and the emphasis on particular topics have not developed randomly. All are based on my long experience with advocacy among nonprofessionals. All of them reflect an intentional way of approaching nonprofessionals for the purposes of mental health education.

For instance, I have avoided arguing with critics of psychiatry, regardless of whether they are internal or external. A debating attitude implies that the content of the information is controversial, when in fact it is established science. Criticisms of psychiatry are lumped together in Chapter 4. At that point in the book, they serve to heighten the "dramatic tension" and increase motivation for a deeper level of knowledge about mental illness. Why do I not begin the book with criticisms of psychiatry? Because the most important way to introduce mental illness (after providing a few definitions) is to show that it relates to everyone. Why should you care about mental illness? Because you or someone you love has experienced mental illness. It matters to you personally, whether or not you knew it in the past. Only people who view mental health as personally relevant will bother to listen attentively to the rest of what we as advocates have to say about mental health.

Therefore, the emphasis of the first part of the book is on epidemiology and the universal significance of mental health.

It would be tedious to detail my reasons for the myriad of other choices behind these pages. You will find it easy enough to evaluate whether they are helpful to your work. I hope that you will not be put off by reading chapters pitched at the level of laypersons rather than professionals. I have attempted to communicate in a way that is straightforward and fast-moving, rather than patronizing or simplistic. I hope that you will read the book from a personal and not merely critical perspective, and that you will experience the fascination, hope, and enthusiasm that I feel when contemplating the extraordinary edifice of science and medicine that stands behind our work. Those of us privileged enough to practice mental health care are among the luckiest people on earth, in my opinion. Our field gives us intellectual fascination, emotional connection, and ethical/existential purpose. And thanks to many decades of research, we can now appreciate that our work addresses the physical, emotional, and social well-being of our patients in real and effective ways. This information—the powerful science supporting our work—should energize and stimulate us, and likewise should energize the public on behalf of those with mental illness. Laid out before us, it should provide more than enough conviction that the time is ripe for cultural transformation and a new era in the treatment of mental health disorders. If it did not, I would be as surprised as I was disappointed. But it will do so, because such information ultimately rests on reality even more than on idealism, hope, and passion.

Advocacy in Action: Argument of the Book

With these preliminaries out of the way, let's begin the "see one" part of the book. I would like to start with a summary of the whole book, so you know exactly where this discussion is going. The following chapters are filled with facts and details, so these paragraphs will give you a sense of the whole. I hope they clearly convey the central thrust of this book: Mental illness is common, real, serious, and treatable.

Chapter 2: What Is Mental Illness? This book is about mental illness. What do I mean by mental illness? I mean a kind of medical illness that is like every other kind of medical illness, with one addition: mental illness is also mental. While we recognize mental illness from mental symptoms, mental illness also has all the characteristic of medical illnesses. *Mental illness is medical illness that primarily affects mental functions.* So when the part of the body that we need for normal moods gets sick, we can have a mood disorder like major depression or bipolar disorder. Or if the part of the body we need for normal memory gets sick, we can have a memory disorder like Alzheimer's dementia, and so on.

Chapter 3: Mental Illness Is Common. Why should you care about mental illness? Mental illness is relevant to you, because it is relevant to all of us. Mental illness affects you personally, either directly and/or indirectly. How do we know? Several large and detailed studies of the U.S. population find stunningly high rates of mental illness. About one in four persons experiences mental illness every year, and more than half the population will do so during a lifetime. Half of all Americans will experience mental illness at some point in life. And statistically, that means either you will be affected yourself or someone you love will be affected. So mental illness concerns you indirectly through people you love, or directly by experiencing it yourself.

Chapter 4: The Myth of Mental Illness? How can so many people have mental illness? Some people do not believe mental illness could be so common. They include doctors, university professors, and even psychiatrists and psychologists. They say that the huge numbers in these studies cannot be real because mental illness is not truly real. Some of them do not believe that mental illness is a physical illness. Others think that we simply do not know whether mental illness is medically real, and accuse doctors of creating definitions of mental illness that suit their own ideas. Finally, some think that while some mental illnesses are probably real, doctors have over-diagnosed and overmedicated people without much justification. But all of them believe that mental health care lacks a medical and scientific foundation.

Chapter 5: Mental Illness Is Real. How do we know that mental illness is medically real? Because the scientific research is clear and definitive. We have countless scientific studies that document the biological reality of mental disorders: Genetic studies show that the risk of mental illness is physically passed down over generations. Head scan studies show dysfunction and deterioration of living brains during episodes of mental illness. We can show that hormones and brain transmitters change during mental illness. Other studies show increased inflammation in the body and brain at the same time. We have all this evidence, and much more.

Chapter 6: Mental Illness Is Serious. There is another way to show that mental illness is real. We can show that mental illness has all the real consequences of any medical illness. As supported by facts in Chapter 6, mental illness is serious. Why do we dread medical illness? We fear death, disability, and deterioration of our health. These three consequences—death, disability, and deterioration—are just as common in mental illness as in other types of medical illness. For instance, suicide (sudden death from mental illness) is the fourth leading cause of death for adults ages 18–65. And mental illness causes people to spend more time in disability than any other kind of illness. Finally, mental illness causes wear and tear on our bodies, increasing our risk of heart disease and other chronic illnesses.

Chapter 7: Mental Illness Is Nobody's Fault. Mental illness is bad news. But there is also some good news. No one is to blame for mental illness. It is not the fault of parents, of mental health professionals, or of the people who have it. Why does this matter? People with mental illness and their families have been blamed, shamed, and abused for centuries. Most people dealing with mental illness have experienced stigma and misunderstanding. So not blaming anyone *is* a big deal. Understanding the real causes of mental illness would be even better, especially because the basic causes of mental illness are simple: genes plus stresses.

Chapter 8: Mental Illness Is Treatable. Everyone knows there are treatments for mental illness, but few people know just how effective these treatments are. Most people know that we cannot (usually) cure mental illness, but most people forget that we cannot usually cure high blood pressure, diabetes, heart disease, or most other chronic illnesses. Yet we can treat them all. And it turns out that treatment for mental illness is generally as good as treatment for other chronic medical conditions. Medicines for mental health are just as likely to work as medicines for other conditions. And on top of medicines, we have powerful and proven treatments such as talk therapy and social supports.

Chapter 9: Mental Illness Is Our Teacher: How can mental illness become our teacher? Mental illness usually begins early in life, when people are teenagers or young adults. Facing chronic illness and limitations as a young person is excruciatingly painful. At the same time, those who do face the realities of illness and limitations in life develop a deep wisdom that we will all need at some point. They have learned how to accept life on its own terms and to find meaning and satisfaction in life despite the presence of pain and adversity. This is a profound understanding of the human condition, and we would all do well to listen and learn from it, because mental illness is just another part of the human condition, every bit as much as illness, aging, and death are.

Chapter 10: A Vision of Unity. Mental illness affects everyone. Sigmund Freud had mental illness, and so have many famous psychiatrists and psychologists of history. Why should we remember this? We should remember that there is really no difference between people with mental illness and everybody else. "They" are not a separate category of persons. "They" are the doctors, the family members, the people with mental illness, the people who love people with mental illness. We are all in the same boat, and the sooner we all realize this, the sooner that boat will go in the right direction.

What is the point of this book? The point is that you or someone you love has had or currently has mental illness. And if you or someone you love has mental illness, it is possible to know and fully experience the following truths with confidence and clarity:

- Mental illness is common: You are not alone.
- Mental illness is real: You are not making this up.
- Mental illness is serious: You are not weak.
- Mental illness is nobody's fault: You are not to blame.
- Mental illness is treatable: There is help.

References

Agency for Healthcare Research and Quality: The number of nurse practitioners and physician assistants practicing primary care in the United States. September 2018a. Available at: www.ahrq.gov/research/findings/factsheets/primary/pcwork2/index.html. Accessed April 19, 2020.

Agency for Healthcare Research and Quality: The number of practicing primary care physicians in the United States. July 2018b. Available at: www.ahrq.gov/research/findings/factsheets/primary/pcwork1/index.html. Accessed April 19, 2020.

American Psychological Association: How many psychologists are licensed in the United States? Monitor on Psychology 45(6):13, 2014. Available at: www.apa.org/monitor/2014/06/datapoint. Accessed April 19, 2020.

American Psychological Association: Survey: Americans becoming more open about mental health. May 2019. Available at: www.apa.org/news/press/releases/apa-mental-health-report.pdf. Accessed April 16, 2020.

American Psychiatric Association: Diagnostic and Statistical Manual of Mental Disorders, 5th Edition. Arlington, VA, American Psychiatric Association, 2013

Appelbaum PS, Parks J: Holding insurers accountable for parity in coverage of mental health treatment. Psychiatr Serv 71(2):202–204, 2020

Banaschewski T, Gerlach M, Becker K, et al: Trust, but verify: the errors and misinterpretations in the Cochrane analysis by OJ Storebo and colleagues on the efficacy and safety of methylphenidate for the treatment of children and adolescents with ADHD. Z Kinder Jugendpsychiatr Psychother 44(4):307–314, 2016

Barsaglini A, Sartori G, Benetti S, et al: The effects of psychotherapy on brain function: a systematic and critical review. Prog Neurobiol 114:1–14, 2014

Bishop TF, Seirup JK, Pincus HA, et al: Population of U.S. practicing psychiatrists declined, 2003–13, which may help explain poor access to mental health care. Health Aff (Millwood) 35(7):1271–1277, 2016

Bloom P: Descartes' Baby: How the Science of Child Development Explains What Makes Us Human. New York, Basic Books, 2005

Brikell I, Kuja-Halkola R, Larsson H: Heritability of attention-deficit hyperactivity disorder in adults. Am J Med Genet B Neuropsychiatr Genet 168(6):406–413, 2015

Carlat D: Unhinged: The Trouble With Psychiatry—A Doctor's Revelations About a Profession in Crisis. New York, Simon & Schuster, 2010

Cooke A (ed): Understanding Psychosis and Schizophrenia. British Psychological Society, Division of Clinical Psychology, 2014. Available at: www.bps.org.uk/what-psychology/understanding-psychosis-and-schizophrenia. Accessed January 4, 2019.

De Pinto J, Backus F: Most Americans think there is stigma associated with mental illness—CBS News poll. CBS News, October 23, 2019. Available at: www.cbsnews.com/news/most-americans-think-there-is-stigma-associated-with-mental-illness-cbs-news-poll. Accessed May 8, 2020.

Fountoulakis KN, Hoschl C, Kasper S, et al: The media and intellectuals' response to medical publications: the antidepressants' case. Ann Gen Psychiatry 12(1):11, 2013

Frances A: The British Psychological Society enters the silly season. Psychiatric Times, May 15, 2013. Available at: www.psychiatrictimes.com/view/british-psychological-society-enters-silly season. Accessed June 12, 2020.

Frances A: What drives our dumb and disorganized policies on mental health? Psychiatric Times, October 9, 2015. Available at: www.psychiatrictimes.com/couch-crisis/what-drives-our-disorganized-mental-health-policies. Accessed May 7, 2020.

Greenberg GA: Psychiatry's incurable hubris. The Atlantic, April 2019, pp 30–32. Available at: www.theatlantic.com/magazine/archive/2019/04/mind-fixers-anne-harrington/583228. Accessed July 30, 2019.

Harrington A: Mind Fixers: Psychiatry's Troubled Search for the Biology of Mental Illness. New York, WW Norton, 2019

Kaiser Permanente: New poll: progress and persistent myths about mental health. October 2, 2017. Available at: https://findyourwords.org/understanding-depression/mental-health-myths-facts-national-poll. Accessed January 8, 2021.

Kendler KS: Toward a philosophical structure for psychiatry. Am J Psychiatry 162(3):433–440, 2005

Leucht S, Hierl S, Kissling W, et al: Putting the efficacy of psychiatric and general medicine medication into perspective: review of meta-analyses. Br J Psychiatry 200(2):97–106, 2012

Lewis M: Brain change in addiction as learning, not disease. N Engl J Med 379(16):1551–1560, 2018

Livingston JD, Boyd JE: Correlates and consequences of internalized stigma for people living with mental illness: a systematic review and meta-analysis. Soc Sci Med 71(12):2150–2161, 2010

Luhrmann TM: Of Two Minds: An Anthropologist Looks at American Psychiatry. New York, Vintage, 2001

McAllister-Williams RH: Do antidepressants work? A commentary on "Initial severity and antidepressant benefits: a meta-analysis of data submitted to the Food and Drug Administration" by Kirsch et al. Evid Based Ment Health 11(3):66–68, 2008

Parcesepe AM, Cabassa LJ: Public stigma of mental illness in the United States: a systematic literature review. Adm Policy Ment Health 40(5):384–399, 2013

Pies R: The war on psychiatric diagnosis. Psychiatric Times, April 3, 2015. Available at: www.psychiatrictimes.com/view/war-psychiatric-diagnosis. Accessed July 21, 2020.

Phillips J, Frances A, Cerullo MA, et al: The six most essential questions in psychiatric diagnosis: a pluralogue part 1: conceptual and definitional issues in psychiatric diagnosis. Philos Ethics Humanit Med 7(1):3, 2012

Prasad V, Vandross A, Toomey C, et al: A decade of reversal: an analysis of 146 contradicted medical practices. Mayo Clin Proc 88(8):790–798, 2013

Research America: Taking our pulse: the PARADE/Research America health poll. Charlton Research Company, 2006. Available at: www.researchamerica.org/sites/default/files/uploads/paradearticlementalhealth1006.pdf. Accessed April 17, 2020.

Sajatovic M, Velligan DI, Weiden PJ, et al: Measurement of psychiatric treatment adherence. J Psychosom Res 69(6):591–599, 2010

Salsberg E, Quigley L, Mehfoud N, et al: Profile of the Social Work Workforce. A Report to Council on Social Work Education and National Workforce Initiative Steering Committee From the George Washington University Health Workforce Institute and School of Nursing. October 2017. Available at: www.cswe.org/Centers-Initiatives/Initiatives/National-Workforce-Initiative/SW-Workforce-Book-FINAL-11-08-2017.aspx. Accessed April 19, 2020.

Stein D: Philosophy of Psychopharmacology. Cambridge, UK, Cambridge University Press, 2008

Substance Abuse and Mental Health Services Administration: Key substance use and mental health indicators in the United States: results from the 2017 National Survey on Drug Use and Health (HHS Publ No SMA-18-5068, NSDUH Series H-53). Rockville, MD, Center for Behavioral Health Statistics and Quality, Substance Abuse and Mental Health Services Administration, 2018. Available at: www.samhsa.gov/data/sites/default/files/cbhsq-reports/NSDUHFFR2017/NSDUHFFR2017.pdf. Accessed July 21, 2020.

Szalai J: Mental illness is all in your brain—or is it? The New York Times. April 24, 2019. Available at: www.nytimes.com/2019/04/24/books/review-mind-fixers-psychiatry-biology-mental-illness-anne-harrington.html. Accessed June 16, 2019.

Torrey EF, Kennard AD, Eslinger D, et al: More Mentally Ill Persons Are in Jails and Prisons Than Hospitals: A Survey of the States. Treatment Advocacy Center, May 2010. Available at: www.treatmentadvocacycenter.org/storage/documents/final_jails_v_hospitals_study.pdf. Accessed July 21, 2020.

Universal Health Services: UHS releases results of poll examining Americans' perceptions on mental health. March 2019. Available at: www.uhsinc.com/uhs-releases-results-of-poll-examining-americans-perceptions-on-mental-health. Accessed April 17, 2020.

U.S. Bureau of Labor Statistics: Occupational employment statistics. Occupational employment and wages, May 2019: 21-1018 Substance abuse, behavioral disorder, and mental health counselors. May 2019. Available at: www.bls.gov/oes/current/oes211018.htm. Accessed April 19, 2020.

Vindegaard N, Benros ME: COVID-19 pandemic and mental health consequences: systematic review of the current evidence. Brain Behav Immun 89:531–542, 2020

Volkow ND, Koob GF, McLellan AT: Neurobiologic advances from the brain disease model of addiction. N Engl J Med 374(4):363–371, 2016

Wang PS, Lane M, Olfson M, et al: Twelve-month use of mental health services in the United States: results from the National Comorbidity Survey Replication. Arch Gen Psychiatry 62(6):629–640, 2005

Woolf SH, Schoomaker H: Life expectancy and mortality rates in the United States, 1959–2017. JAMA 322(20):1996–2016, 2019

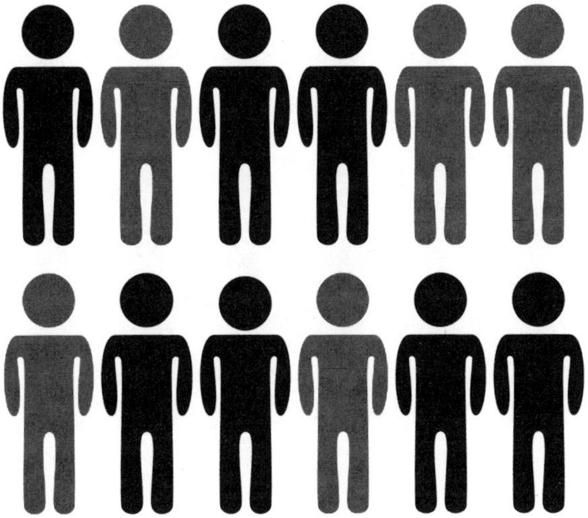

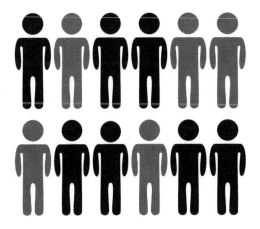

What Is Mental Illness?

Half Truth: Mental illness is mental or physical.
Whole Truth: Mental illness is mental and physical.

Important Points

- Mental illness is a kind of medical illness.
- Medical illness is physical dysfunction causing distress.
- Mental illness is medical illness that shows itself mainly through mental symptoms.
- All mental symptoms correspond to brain activity.
- Since the brain is the most complex object in the universe, mental illness is unimaginably complex and very difficult to understand.

Introduction

Definitions generally bore people, and rightly so. Any complex abstract discussion about the nature of mental life and mental illness is likely to lose a discussion partner straightaway. However, there are so many pervasive misconceptions about mental illness that we as advocates cannot begin to speak of it without some basic clarifications. Some people understand *mental illness* as referring only to severe and disabling forms of illness such as schizophrenia; they can only imagine someone with mental illness as an unkempt person who is homeless. Others take mental illness to refer to all manner of stress and inner pain, making times of normal human sadness into depression and normal human stress into anxiety disorders. So any discussion of mental illness must begin with some brief effort to clarify what we are talking about.

Two clarifications are most important here: First, mental illness is unambiguously medical, physical, and biological. This statement refers to the physical dysfunction that characterizes all medical illness, and not merely mental anguish or even troubles with mental functioning. Second, mental illness is unambiguously mental and psychological. Mental illness primarily expresses itself by altering mental functions. Thus, we begin with the fundamental assertion that there is no difference between the biological and the psychological in regard to mental illness and its treatment. The two are always present in mental illness. They do not exclude or compete with each other.

The most concise way to present this sort of holism is through the biopsychosocial model, or, if you and your audience are so inclined, the biopsychosocial-spiritual model. This approach has an intuitive and universal appeal that rapidly allows laypersons to grasp that we are not proposing any sort of reductionism. Note that I am not using the biopsychosocial model as a model here, or as a paradigm, or as a conceptual framework. I am using it as a mnemonic, to remind us and our listeners that the reality of a human being exists at multiple levels of increasing complexity, and that all of these levels are relevant for understanding mental health and mental illness. In other words, I am adopting (what I believe to be) the general consensus view of human nature in psychiatry and neuroscience: Psychological and social levels of human experience exist biologically, but they are so complex that we cannot currently describe them in concise and coherent biological terms. At the same time, these higher levels of complexity are causally real, both in instigating and in relieving mental illness. Therefore, biological, psychological, and social factors are all "real" and necessary for both understanding and addressing mental illness (Kendler 2005).

A Note of Respect for the Human Brain

Mental illness afflicts the human brain, and the human brain is the most complex object in the physical universe. There is no physical thing in the universe more highly coordinated or extensively organized than the thing you carry around inside your own head. It consists of approximately 100 billion neurons (Herculano-Houzel 2009). Each of these neurons connects with ten to 30,000 other neurons (Megías et al. 2001). Nerve cells (at least on the brain's cortical surface) each connect with an average of 7,000 other nerve cells (Drachman 2005), making for a possible 0.5–1 quadrillion connections between brain neurons. Hypothetically, we could say that there are more possible brain states than there are atoms in the universe (Edelman 1992). The human brain has no serious competition: It is *the* wonder of the known universe.

This book is about the human brain, but it is not only about the human brain. The brain is at the center of who you are as a human being, but it is the *hub* of who you are, not the *whole* of who you are. Your brain is intimately interconnected with every system in your body, it is intimately connected with your interior psychological world, and it is intimately interconnected with the world around you. You are so much more than just the physical aspect of your brain, and all this complexity is what makes mental illness possible.

Even by itself, the human brain is unimaginably complicated. We should all be in awe that the brain, having 100 billion "moving parts," works at all. How is it even possible that with hundreds of trillions of connections, we are able to walk and chew gum at the same time? How is it possible that we can even walk? And if you think walking is easy, ask a few robot engineers, who are painfully aware that decades of research have not produced robots able to walk like human beings (Walker 2019) (Figure 2–1).

Because mental functions involved in mental illness are far more complicated than walking, no one should assume that problems in mental function are unusual among human beings. Problems are common, and they are not a sign of weakness. Instead, they are a sign of the literally unthinkable complexity of being human. With trillions of interconnections, no one should be surprised that brains can break down on a regular basis. And no one should think organs so complicated would not be subject to illness. Every organ in the body is subject to breakdowns. The more complicated the organ, the more possible things can go wrong. The brain is by far the most complicated organ in the body, and there are more ways for the brain to break down than for any other organ.

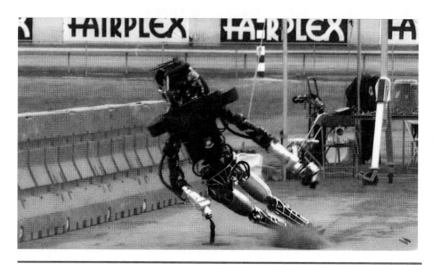

FIGURE 2–1. Walking—not as easy as it looks.

Source.   Video still from "DARPA: DARPA Robotics Challenge Finals: A Celebration of Risk." June 6, 2015. Available at: https://archive.darpa.mil/roboticschallenge/gallery-all.html. Accessed July 22, 2020.

What Is Medical Illness?

Mental illness occurs when the brain breaks down. But the brain is only one of many organs in the body, and mental illness is only one of many types of medical illness. So we need to talk about medical illness before we try to define mental illness. Medical illness is *a physical dysfunction that causes distress.* Thus, there are two parts to medical conditions, sometimes divided into dysfunction and harm (Wakefield 2007), or disease and illness (Boyd 2000). Disease is the part about physical dysfunction—the body is not working the way it is supposed to work. Distress (illness or harm) is about the human experience of being unwell, and often includes both suffering and the inability to function normally; that is, we feel bad and we cannot do what we would normally do. For our purposes, we will use "illness" for both the dysfunction and the distress. So, for instance, when you are ill with the flu, viruses are invading and disrupting your respiratory system (dysfunction), while you feel feverish, achy, tired, and unable to get out of bed (distress). Mental illness is just a form of physical illness, so mental illness also involves physical dysfunction and human distress.

What Is Mental Illness?

Mental illness is a kind of medical illness. It is the same as every other kind of medical illness (Wakefield 1992). Mental illness involves just as much physical dysfunction and just as much distress as any other type of medical illness (see Chapters 5 and 6). It differs from other medical illnesses in only one respect: *Mental illness is the type of medical illness that mainly affects mental functions.* More precisely, mental illness is the type of medical illness that primarily affects parts of the brain that we need for mental functions. For instance, when the part of the brain that we need for normal mood gets sick, we can have a mood disorder like major depression or bipolar (manic-depressive) disorder. Or if the part of the brain that we need for normal fear gets sick, we can have an anxiety disorder like panic attacks or posttraumatic stress disorder (PTSD). Finally, if the part of the brain we need for normal memory gets sick, we can have a memory disorder like Alzheimer's dementia. Figure 2–2 lists some common mental illnesses.

Like medical illness, mental illness requires both bodily dysfunction and an experience of distress—that is suffering and/or being unable to function. Put briefly, mental illness means that the brain is not functioning normally, and we either feel bad or cannot do what we normally would. Someone with severe depression, for instance, feels horrible emotional pain inside, while being unable to do things like get out of bed or take a shower. Finally, what makes mental illness mental is that it is, well, mental. It affects our normal ways of perceiving the world, thinking, feeling, deciding, and acting. At least some of these abilities will be affected by a mental illness. So mental illness involves everything we see in medical illness, but on top of that mental illness affects our mental functions.

Is Mental Illness Mental or Physical?

For centuries, people have debated the nature of mental illness. There have always been some who said it was physical and others who said it was mental. Today, we finally have a clear answer: *Mental illness is both.* The rest of the book will expand on this answer, but it is important for all of us to get out of the either/or mindset once and for all. Human beings are mental, and we are also physical. The mind is mental, and the brain is physical. Being human means having both, and having both means we are able to function as human

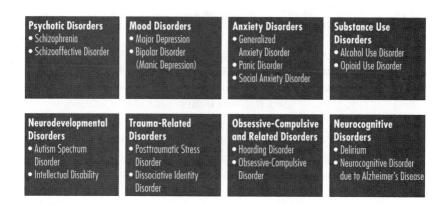

Psychotic Disorders	Mood Disorders	Anxiety Disorders	Substance Use Disorders
• Schizophrenia • Schizoaffective Disorder	• Major Depression • Bipolar Disorder (Manic Depression)	• Generalized Anxiety Disorder • Panic Disorder • Social Anxiety Disorder	• Alcohol Use Disorder • Opioid Use Disorder
Neurodevelopmental Disorders	Trauma-Related Disorders	Obsessive-Compulsive and Related Disorders	Neurocognitive Disorders
• Autism Spectrum Disorder • Intellectual Disability	• Posttraumatic Stress Disorder • Dissociative Identity Disorder	• Hoarding Disorder • Obsessive-Compulsive Disorder	• Delirium • Neurocognitive Disorder due to Alzheimer's Disease

FIGURE 2–2. Examples of mental illnesses.

This figure lists some common or commonly mentioned examples of mental illness. Many more mental illnesses are detailed in the *Diagnostic and Statistical Manual of Mental Disorders*, 5th Edition (DSM-5; American Psychiatric Association 2013).

beings. When illness affects our mental functions, illness simultaneously affects our physical lives as well. If it did not do both, it would not be mental illness. Happily, the name "mental illness" tells us all we need to know. It is "mental" and affects the nonphysical parts of who we are, while at the same time it is physical "illness" and affects the bodily part of who we are.

What Is a Human Being?

The realization that mental illness is both mental and physical only brings up a deeper question: How is it that human beings are both mental and physical? How is it possible that "I" can have internal, mental thoughts, feelings and imaginings that no one else can see or sense, at the same time feel like "I" inhabit a body, and at the same time feel that "I" *am* my body? Well today, after centuries of debate and investigation, we now have an answer. Philosophers, brain scientists, psychologists, and psychiatrists generally agree: We do not know. We do not know how human beings are both mental and physical. We only know that we *are* both mental and physical and that the mental and physical are intimately intertwined. Our brain cells, neurotransmitters, hormones, immune system, and even gut bacteria affect our mental lives. At the same time, our thoughts, mental habits, feelings, and ways of perceiving the world deeply affect our bodies, including our hormones, our immune system, and even our gut bacteria. Mind affects body, and body affects mind. We know this, even if we do not understand how.

Mind and body are no longer seen as mutually exclusive. We no longer say, "This problem is mental, therefore it is not physical." Instead, we say that mind and body (or mind and brain) are two sides of the same coin. They go together, hand in hand. They are best friends that you always see together, not two rivals in competition with each other. So today, when we find that we can treat mental illness with medications, we do not say, "Aha! Medicines and biological therapies work, so talk therapy and mental treatments don't!" It turns out that these medicines have both biological and psychological effects, just like talk therapies have both biological and psychological effects (Chapter 8). Mind affects body, and body affects mind. More precisely, mind/body are two aspects of one thing (Kendler 2005).

All of this brings us closer to an idea of what it means to be a human being: To be a human being is to be one thing with different aspects. Mind and body are two aspects of who we are, but they are not all of who we are. We are more than an individual body and an individual, internal mind. How many dimensions or aspects are there to a human being? Probably as many as we would like to name. Yet for the purposes of mental health, we typically name four aspects of being human: biological, psychological, social, and spiritual. This is sometimes called the *biopsychosocial-spiritual model* (see Engel 1980; Hiatt 1986).

Why do we include social and spiritual factors? Because social and spiritual factors also profoundly affect our mental and physical health. For instance, scientific studies have shown that social support is a powerful factor in promoting physical and mental health. So much so that a lack of social support seems to be as bad for physical health as smoking (see Chapter 8). Spiritual factors also influence physical and mental health. For instance, spiritual practices such as meditation or attending religious services are associated with better immune function, lower levels of inflammation, and a longer, healthier life (see Chapter 8).

One other note about the biopsychosocial-spiritual model: These four aspects of life are not parts that go together to build a human being. Instead, they represent different points of view as we look at the same human being. We cannot ultimately detach the spiritual from the physical, or the social from the psychological. Therefore, we could define being human in this way: *A human being is a person with biological, psychological, social, and spiritual dimensions.*

What does all of this have to do with mental illness? First, if we no longer have to decide whether mental illness is mental or physical, then we no longer have to debate about whether to use a physical treatment like medicine for mental illness. Many people tend to feel guilty about taking a medicine for a mental illness like panic disorder, as if it is a sign of weakness. This implies that people who are mentally strong can simply control their own thoughts and not be anxious. And this, in turn, implies a mental illness like anxiety is not physical. If thoughts are just mental, we should be able to control them. And yet most people do not feel the same way about taking a medicine for blood pressure or an ear infection because these are physical. We do not expect to fully control the body with our minds, and we feel fine about using physical medicines for our physical bodies. So if mental illness is physical as well as mental, then it is very straightforward to take a medicine for the physical part of mental illness. No guilt is required.

Second, if mental illness is both physical and mental, scientifically proven mental treatments like psychotherapy ("talk therapy") are also appropriate. People should not be given a hard time for getting psychotherapy if they suffer from a mental illness. Talk therapy is not psychobabble, and I am going to show some evidence for this later. We will also look at scientific evidence that social treatments (like Alcoholics Anonymous) are powerful, and that even spiritual practices can have mental and physical benefits (Chapter 8). Why is this so? Because human beings are one thing with mental, physical, social and spiritual aspects. When it comes to mental illness, all are relevant. All of these factors affect each other. All are involved with mental illness, and all are involved in mental health (Kendler 2005; Walter 2013).

For a long time, psychiatry was divided by people who believed in the biological side of mental illness, and people who believed in the psychological side (Carlat 2010; Luhrmann 2001). People who believed that mental illnesses were biological thought that medicine was the most appropriate treatment, and that talk therapy might be beside the point. People who believed that mental illnesses were psychological thought that talk therapy was the appropriate treatment, and that medicines might be harmful and unnecessary. In similar fashion, some critics outside of psychiatry have said that mental illness is just a "social construct," something made up by psychiatrists and psychologists that did not reflect biological and psychological realities (Scheff 1966). They asserted that other cultures might not have any mental illness because they had different cultural understandings of people who are different or "deviant." And finally, there have been people outside of psychiatry who have said that there is no mental illness because symptoms of mental illness all reflect spiritual problems, from demon possession to lack of faith (Koenig 2000; Stanford 2012).

But all were wrong whenever they insisted that mental illness was only biological or psychological or social or spiritual. It is "all of the above," because being human involves all of these. Mental illness involves all aspects of being human, and so does its treatment. I am happy to say that the days of such deep splits about mental health are coming to an end (Kandel 1998). The days of never-ending, fruitless debates over these issues are coming to an end. The days of confusing and discouraging people with mental illness (and their families) with such debates are coming to an end. And they are not coming back. Who says so? Science says so. So let's look at the science of mental illness.

Advice for Advocacy

- It is important to demonstrate respect for your audience or conversation partners from the beginning. As a mental health or medical professional, you bring a special expertise, but patients, families, and longtime advocates bring their own significant expertise to these encounters. Acknowledging this from the beginning goes a long way toward making alliances.

- If you can use visual aids such as PowerPoint, use them. Minimize text and maximize use of pictures. Include not only graphs but also illustrative or evocative pictures related to the content of your presentation. Funny and cute pictures can be effective. Remember, you are not trying to convey the most information but rather to engage and energize your audience.

- You may spend very little time discussing definitions in a brief or less technical discussion. For instance, you may define *mental illness* as "the kind of medical illness that causes mental symptoms," give a few examples, and move on.

- Practically speaking, you only need terms and definitions to orient your audience. You do not need definitions to be airtight, and you are not attempting to prove anything through the use of definitions and concepts. For example, defining *mental illness* as being both mental and physical avoids misunderstandings, but it doesn't prove that mental illness is both mental and physical. Only scientific evidence does so.

- There is no generally accepted scientific theory of consciousness. This means that you are under no pressure to supply one. However, understanding mental illness and its treatment does require some type of acceptance that brain and mind are "two sides of the same coin."

- While it is important to insist that mental and physical dimensions are real and not in competition, you can also offer a "big tent" to include people who tend toward religious beliefs (in the immortal soul), those who lean toward biological reductionism (more precisely, epiphenomenalism), and those who lean toward social constructions of mental illness.

References

American Psychiatric Association: Diagnostic and Statistical Manual of Mental Disorders, 5th Edition. Arlington, VA, American Psychiatric Association, 2013

Boyd KM: Disease, illness, sickness, health, healing and wholeness: exploring some elusive concepts. Med Humanit 26(1):9–17, 2000

Carlat D: Unhinged: The Trouble With Psychiatry—A Doctor's Revelations About a Profession in Crisis. New York, Simon & Schuster, 2010

Drachman DA: Do we have brain to spare? Neurology 64(12):2004–2005, 2005

Edelman GM: Bright Air, Brilliant Fire: On the Matter of the Mind. New York, Basic Books, 1992

Engel GL: The clinical application of the biopsychosocial model. Am J Psychiatry 137(5):535–544, 1980

Herculano-Houzel S: The human brain in numbers: a linearly scaled-up primate brain. Front Hum Neurosci 3:31, 2009

Hiatt JF: Spirituality, medicine, and healing. South Med J 79(6):736–743, 1986

Kandel ER: A new intellectual framework for psychiatry. Am J Psychiatry 155(4):457–569, 1998

Kendler KS: Toward a philosophical structure for psychiatry. Am J Psychiatry 162(3):433–440, 2005

Koenig HG: Religion and medicine I: historical background and reasons for separation. Int J Psychiatry Med 30(4):385–398, 2000

Luhrmann TM: Of Two Minds: An Anthropologist Looks at American Psychiatry. New York, Vintage, 2001

Megías M, Emri ZS, Freund TF, et al: Total number and distribution of inhibitory and excitatory synapses on hippocampal CA1 pyramidal cells. Neuroscience 102(3):527–540, 2001

Scheff TJ: Being Mentally Ill: A Sociological Theory. Chicago, IL, Aldine, 1966

Stanford MS: Grace for the Afflicted: A Clinical and Biblical Perspective on Mental Illness. Downers Grove, IL, InterVarsity Press, 2012

Wakefield JC: The concept of mental disorder: on the boundary between biological facts and social values. Am Psychol 47(3):373–388, 1992

Wakefield JC: The concept of mental disorder: diagnostic implications of the harmful dysfunction analysis. World Psychiatry 6(3):149–156, 2007

Walker J: Biped robot timelines—how long until robots move like humans? Emerj Artificial Intelligence Research, February 3, 2019. Available at: https://emerj.com/ai-adoption-timelines/biped-robot-timelines. Accessed July 22, 2020.

Walter H: The third wave of biological psychiatry. Front Psychol 4:582, 2013

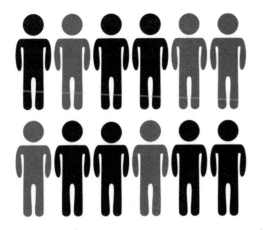

Mental Illness Is Common

Half Truth: Mental illness affects a lot of people.
Whole Truth: Mental illness affects all people.

Important Points

- About one-fourth of the American population experiences mental illness each year.
- About half of the American population experiences mental illness in their lifetime.
- In any year, more people experience mental illness than get the flu.
- In a lifetime, your odds of having mental illness are about the same as your odds of being a woman (or a man).
- Mental illness affects everyone, either directly or indirectly through someone you love.

- Mood disorders, anxiety disorders, and substance use disorders are the most common types of mental illness.
- Psychotic disorders like schizophrenia are the most severe and disabling mental disorders.

Introduction

The most important fact about mental illness is that it affects everyone. If we as advocates convey this one reality to the general public, the political and social calculus of mental health will forever change. Overnight, the second-class status of mental health care will become unacceptable. Mental illness will become everyone's issue, as indeed it is. But the urgency of this fact cannot be communicated through general assertions. Mental health only becomes important as individual people realize that their own family members, their own friends, and their own close coworkers are affected by it. It becomes important when people grasp that the majority of people they know will experience mental illness during their lifetime. Mental health becomes important when it becomes personal, when it becomes a matter of "us" and not just "them."

Happily, we have the science to prove that mental illness is very common. The epidemiology of psychiatric disorders in the United States is exceptionally well developed. Beginning with the Epidemiologic Catchment Area study in the 1980s (Regier et al. 1984), along with others documented in this chapter, we have been given an extraordinarily accurate picture of mental illness in America. These studies involve many thousands of subjects, validated screening and diagnostic instruments, extensive interviews, and careful reviews by teams of experts. They consistently show that vast numbers of people experience significant mental illness every year, people of every demographic and community.

One final note that I believe to be of substantial significance: The commonly repeated point that 1 in 5 Americans suffers mental illness every year is likely to be an understatement. This number should probably be 1 in 4. I believe that the 1 in 5 number is derived from the large, annual SAMHSA survey. However, substance use disorders are reported separately from mental health disorders in this study. If we combine these two categories (taking substance use disorders as mental illnesses), approximately 24% suffer an episode of mental illness in any given year, consistent with the National Comorbidity Surveys (Table 3–1). One in 4 persons suffers an episode of mental illness every year. Mental illness is common, by any conceivable standard. And given the number, size, and quality of the studies behind it, this assertion may be the best supported in all of psychiatry. We should not be shy about articulating it.

Mental Illness: Does Anyone Share the News?

As human beings, we all want to put our best foot forward. Social psychologists have confirmed what common sense tells us: We want to be seen for the good and competent people that we are, and we make great efforts to show ourselves in that light (Greenwald 1980; Leary 2019). We see these efforts relentlessly on social media: People broadcast their big successes, their children's accomplishments, their wonderful relationships, their beauty, their possessions, their social lives. They do so day after day after day, at times advertising themselves like corporations. If you go on social media right now, you will find that one of your friends just finished the best breakfast of his life! Another will show you just how much her husband loves her! Another has a child who just graduated from Harvard! Then an acquaintance will show pictures of his fabulous dream vacation to Hawaii.

We all want to feel good about ourselves, to feel that others like and admire us. Some of us are just more overt about it than others. Also, all of us feel embarrassed about our failures or weaknesses, and most of us try to hide these from ourselves and others. This is part of human nature. It is not at all surprising, then, that most people do go not around broadcasting their recent experiences with mental illness. Most people do not post on social media about being suicidal (though some do), and most people do not go around wearing buttons that say, "Hug me, I have mental illness." None of us will ever see "overcame major depression" on someone's resume, and there will never be a "Person of the Year" award for "best job fighting schizophrenia." After all, mental illness tends to feel like personal weakness (Kaiser Permanente 2018), and although our culture is increasingly accepting of mental illness, stigma persists (Parcesepe and Cabassa 2013). There is nothing wrong with the fact that people do not publicly trumpet the pain, struggle, and disappointment of dealing with mental illness. Health matters are private, and no one should feel guilty for not sharing. The choice of whether or not to share is personal.

Because people do not often talk about it, none of us gets a direct impression of how common or unusual mental illness might be. Those who have not suffered from mental illness might be forgiven for the vague emotional impression that it is unusual, and for assuming that mental health problems are the exception rather than the rule. Even if you know that mental illness is common, you might not see it affect the people around you very much. After all, people who post on social media seem to be doing just fine. And people you encounter regularly may not talk about it much. Thus, mental illness often ends up affecting other people instead of the people around you. If you do not experience mental illness yourself, then mental conditions seem to affect "those people," people who are different from you, rather than affecting "us people," the people who are part of your life.

For people actually dealing with mental illness the situation is even more confusing. If you or someone in your family deals with mental illness, you find yourself quickly feeling isolated and inferior, as if you are failing and falling behind in the great race of life. From personal experience, I can say the same thing as many others in this position: Without even thinking about it, you desperately try to avoid letting anyone know. People ask you how you are and after an unconvincing "pretty good," you steer the conversation in another direction. You carry a secret load of sadness and pain 24 hours a day, either for yourself or someone you love. People ask what is wrong and you say things like, "I'm just tired today." But you feel dead inside—that is, when you don't feel terrified. It is impossible to feel good about yourself. Instead, you are just hoping that no one will see what is going on inside you and your private life. Mental illness makes people feel as if they are on the sidelines of life while everyone else is in the middle of a rousing game. It makes people feel inferior, left out, miserable, and even subhuman. All of this plays into the sense that everyone else is doing great and going places in life, and you alone with your mental health problems are not. And this plays into the sense that not many people have to deal with mental illness, even when you know that is not the truth.

So if you deal with mental illness it feels like very few people have it, and if you do not deal with mental illness it often feels like very few people have it. Either way, mental illness does not feel common. And yet our feelings do not match well with what we know. We know that many people do experience mental health conditions. So let's look at what the scientific data tell us and see exactly how many people deal with mental illness.

How Common Is Mental Illness?

Mental Illness Over the Lifetime

Having mental illness is isolating. It feels profoundly lonely. The experience feels profoundly lonely. Yet strangely enough, if you have had mental illness during your lifetime, you are not really in a minority. Far from being alone, you have countless millions for company. The percentage of people who have suffered from mental illness in their lifetime is so large, in fact, that it equals nearly half of the country's population (Table 3–1 and Figure 3–1): An astounding 46%–50% of Americans have already experienced some form of mental illness in their lifetimes, and more than half (55%) will experience it at some time in life (Kessler et al. 2007). Though it is hard to imagine that mental illness is so common, this fact is scientifically solid and well-grounded. So remember this if you remember nothing else: *Mental illness directly affects half of all people over the course of a lifetime.*

If we break down the numbers, we find that anxiety disorders, mood disorders, and substance use disorders are all quite common (Table 3–2). At some point in life, about 1 in 5 persons has had a mood disorder (such as major depression), and 1 in 4 has had a substance use or anxiety disorder. (The next time you are waiting in a crowded room, count the people around you and think about those percentages.) Meanwhile, disorders involving psychosis are much less common but typically much more disabling. Psychosis is a brain dysfunction that makes an individual unable to distinguish the real from the unreal, with symptoms such as hallucinations—seeing things and hearing things that others do not. About 3.5% of the population has experienced psychosis at some point, and around 1% of the population suffers from schizophrenia, a devastating and frequently disabling illness (Perälä et al. 2007). Schizophrenia and other psychotic disorders are not as common as some other mental illnesses, but they are important medical causes of long-term disability.

Of course, these percentages do *not* mean that half the country's population suffers from mental illness right now. They do *not* mean that half the people are constantly ill or that half are disabled by mental illness. When people hear about mental illness, many think of the worst and longest-lasting kinds of mental illness, and understandably cannot believe that half the country could be so affected. Indeed, half of the population is not disabled or overwhelmed by mental illness. Many people have mild forms of mental illness and get through them without any medical treatment at all, just as they do with a bad back or recurrent headaches. Having any mental illness during one's lifetime could include a couple of months of major depression in midlife, or a year of problem drinking (alcohol use disorder) in young adulthood. Sometimes mental illness appears, disappears in a matter of months, and never returns. So this big number (50%) reflects the lifetime risk of any mental illness, not how many people have it today.

What *do* these high percentages mean? They mean, quite simply, that mental illness affects everyone. Mental health disorders affect half the population directly, and they affect everyone else indirectly. This is a statistical certainty. With 50% of the population affected, everyone else is close to someone who has had mental illness. Everyone has a family member, close friend, or close co-worker who is or has been affected by mental illness. Someone you love has had mental illness. How do I know? Because saying you do not know someone who has had mental illness is statistically the same thing as saying you do not know

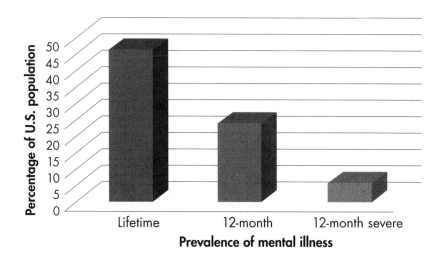

FIGURE 3–1. Prevalence of mental illness.
Source. Data from the National Comorbidity Survey Replication (Kessler et al. 2005a, 2005b).

anyone who is a woman or anyone who is a man. You *do* know someone, but you may not be aware of it. In the case of mental illness, you may not know the other person has had it, because most people do not talk about it, and you cannot tell by looking. But you can be sure that people you know and people you love have had mental illness, whether they are family members or friends. And because mental illness affects half of us, it affects all of us.

This large number also tells us something else. It tells us that you and I can walk into any room, with any group of people under any circumstances, and be confident that mental illness is relevant to those people. Enter a room full of strangers, and you can be certain that they too are affected by mental illness. They too have suffered. Some of them have been through it themselves, and the rest are close to others who have experienced it. Everyone is affected by mental illness, and there are no groups exempt from mental health conditions. Mental illness affects women and men from all ethnic groups, all cultures, all nations, and all age groups. All people are affected, regardless of whether they reside in rural or urban areas and whether they are rich or poor. The most powerful politicians have been affected (Kennedy and Fried 2016; Shenk 2006), as have some of the most successful actors, writers, and artists (Jamison 1996). CEOs have been affected (Dittmann 2005), and so have doctors, lawyers, engineers, and scientists. There are no exceptions. Remember this one reality of mental illness, and I suspect it will energize you as it has me: Mental illness affects us all.

TABLE 3–1. Percentages of U.S. population with mental illness, as reported in large national studies

Study	Lifetime rate	12-month rate	12-month serious mental illness rate	Number of adult participants
NCS	49.7%	30.9%	—	8,098
NCS-R	46.4%	26.2%	5.8%	9,282
NESARC	—	—	—	34,653
NSDUH	—	24.0%	4.5%	50,999

Note. NCS=National Comorbidity Survey (Kessler et al. 1994, 1997); NCS-R=National Comorbidity Survey Replication (Kessler et al. 2005a, 2005b); NESARC=National Epidemiologic Survey on Alcohol and Related Conditions (Hasin and Grant 2015); NSDUH=National Survey on Drug Use and Health (Substance Abuse and Mental Health Services Administration 2018a).

Mental Illness Each Year

Even if we only look at cases of mental illness during the past year, the numbers are still astonishing: According to the best evidence, *in any one year, 24%–31% of Americans experience mental illness* (see Table 3–1). That is about 1 in every 4 persons. One in every 4 people you see driving down the street or at the grocery store knows the pain of mental illness, this year alone.

How common is that? Let's compare it to a common medical problem, like the flu. In any given year, 3%–20% of the population will get the flu (Centers for Disease Control and Prevention 2019). Nobody wants the flu, but it is considered a "normal" or common thing to be sick with the flu. Well, in any given year, more people are going to have mental illness than have the flu. Even in a really bad year for the flu, it is more common, more "normal," to have mental illness. And it should be no more surprising. In truth, there is nothing strange about having an episode of mental illness, any more than it is strange to get the flu in the winter. Both are part of the human experience.

Again, this does not mean that 1 in 4 persons has overwhelming, disabling mental illness this year. That number is around 4%–6% of the general population. The majority of cases of mental illness are mild to moderate, just like most cases of diabetes or high blood pressure. Most cases of most medical illnesses are not severe, and mental illness is the same way. About 1 in 4 cases of mental illness is serious or severe. Still, 4%–6% of the general population experiences severe impairment from mental illness every year (Table 3–1).

TABLE 3–2. Lifetime and 12-month prevalence rates of common mental disorders

Study	Anxiety disorders		Mood disorders		Substance use disorders	
	Lifetime	12-month	Lifetime	12-month	Lifetime	12-month
NCS	19.2%	11.8%	14.7%	8.5%	35.4%	16.1%
NCS-R	28.8%	18.1%	20.8%	19.5%	14.6%	3.8%
NESARC	23.6%	15.6%	17.6%	8.1%	32.3%	9.4%
NSDUH	—	—	—	7.1%[a]	—	7.7%

NCS=National Comorbidity Survey (Kessler et al. 1994, 1997); NCS-R=National Comorbidity Survey Replication (Kessler et al. 2005a, 2005b); NESARC=National Epidemiologic Survey on Alcohol and Related Conditions (Hasin and Grant 2015); NSDUH=National Survey on Drug Use and Health (Substance Abuse and Mental Health Services Administration 2018a). [a]Major depression only; no other mood disorders reported.

About 1 in every 20 persons is seriously impaired by mental illness at this moment. *About 4%–6% of the general population experiences severe impairment from mental illness every year* (Table 3–1). This is a significant number and indicates a major public health concern. How do we wrap our minds around this? Compare it to the fact that about 6% of the U.S. population is under age 5 years (U.S. Census Bureau 2020). Do you know any young children? I would guess that you know a number of children under age 5. I would bet that you see them wherever you go. And you are nearly as likely to know and see people who have serious mental illness, even though you may not know that they have mental illness at all. The extent of this public health crisis represents a challenge that concerns every one of us, every bit as much as the welfare of preschool children concerns every one of us. But almost 5% of our population deals with it, and that represents a major public health crisis. It represents a challenge that concerns every one of us, every bit as much as the welfare of preschool children concerns every one of us.

Let me add a final note about these statistics: The usual number that we hear in public forums is that 1 in 5 persons (20% of the population) experiences mental illness in any year, not 1 in 4 (25%). While I personally have no objection to the 1 in 5 number, I believe that 1 in 4 is a more accurate estimate, for the following reasons: The 1 in 5 number comes from a national study conducted every year by the U.S. government (Substance Abuse and Mental Health Services Administration 2018a). In 2017, 18.9% of the population had "any mental illness," and the number has tended to be a little under 20% of the population per year in this series of studies. That is why many public service announcements tell us that 1 in 5 persons suffers from mental illness every year. However, this 18.9% ("any mental illness") does not include people who have substance use disorders only, with no other kind of mental illness. In 2017, that was 4.2% of the population (10.2 million people). So adding those with only substance use disorders (4.2%) to the rest (18.9%) gives us a total of 24.1% of the population, a number close to other large national studies (Table 3–1). This is about 1 in 4 persons, and for now I believe it is the most likely estimate for the U.S. population.

Is Mental Illness Becoming More Common?

One in 2 persons will suffer from mental illness in their lifetime, 1 in 4 every year. These numbers are vast, representing over 150 million and 75 million Americans, respectively. How do we make sense of this? When faced with such massive numbers, many people start wondering if mental illness has always been so prevalent. Did previous generations suffer from widespread mental illness? We certainly hear a lot more about mental health conditions now, and we heard a lot less about them in the past. In the past, people most certainly did not discuss their own or family member's mental health problems. The stigma was overwhelming, the shame was too great, and people did not "burden" each other with personal problems anyway. It is slowly becoming more acceptable to talk about them, and this makes it even harder to get a sense of how common mental illness was in the past.

The short answer is that we do not know whether mental illness is becoming more common. We did not have the same tools to diagnose and survey people who lived in previous generations. In recent decades, some researchers have detected a trend toward a greater prevalence of conditions such as major depression and autism (Hidaka 2012; Matson and Kozlowski 2011). On the other hand, the evidence is quite debatable, and many are understandably skeptical about a significant increase in rates (Pies 2015).

As a matter of opinion, I am not certain that mental illness was a great deal less common in the *recent* past. Certainly, life has changed drastically during the past hundred years, so anything is possible. But as a psychiatrist, I hear many stories suggesting that parents, grandparents, and even great-grandparents experienced mental illness that was never recognized for what it was. For instance, I know one woman whose mother would get in a mood, go to her room, and literally not come out or speak to anyone for several months at a time. I know a man whose father would get manic, go on spending sprees, run away from home, and eventually crash into depression in a hotel room with bottles of liquor and not much else. I know many people who had a "crazy uncle" who was never able to work, or who had a relative who came back from war unable to function mentally ever again. All of these reports likely describe serious mental illness, yet none of those family members were ever diagnosed or treated. In fact, most families did not even speak of those problems among themselves. The elephant was in the room, and everyone knew not to say one word about it.

However, these kinds of stories only take us back about 100 years, to the time that mental health treatment became more common. What about the time prior to this? Psychiatry only emerged as a medical specialty in the late 1800s, at the same time that other important medical practices like anesthesia for surgery and washing hands to avoid infections emerged. Before this, life was unimaginably different. There were no antibiotics or other effective medicines, and surgery had to be done without anesthesia. Women often died in childbirth, and children frequently did not survive to adulthood. In those times, infections and poor nutrition killed most people. War, plague, and famine were recurrent parts of life. Medically speaking, people lived in a different world, one in which mental illness may not have been as important and heart disease, cancer, and diabetes—our major public health problems today—were not the biggest killers. These chronic illnesses seem to have become more common and important because of changes in our life conditions (Omran 1971). Mental illness may also fall into this category of chronic illnesses that have become more common as people live longer in modern environments (Keyes 2007). So, like diabetes and heart disease, mental illness may be much more common and important now than in the distant past. But we do not know for sure.

In one sense, it seems strange that mental illness has not declined in recent times: Our nation and the world have become more prosperous and safer than previously in history, and life (for most people) seems less harsh than it used to be (Pinker 2012). Why has there not been less stress and less mental illness to go along with it? As I think back about the lives of my parents and grandparents, it seems to me that life is generally easier than it used to be. The relentless physical labor and grinding poverty of past centuries have certainly eased for people in developed countries. Yet paradoxically, life has become both easier and more stressful. Although most of us have it easy compared to our ancestors, the pace of life has undoubtedly increased. Our brains suffer a barrage of overstimulation every day from radios, televisions, computers, smartphones, phone calls, advertising, web searches, email, social media, text messages—the list keeps getting longer. We have far more information to process than any previous generation, and our brains were simply not made for this. The stress is taking a toll on our social systems as well as our nervous systems, and it may be contributing to mental illness. There are certainly some people who think so, according to large surveys and some other studies. For instance, national surveys have shown that since the advent of smartphones in 2007, teenagers (who use them the most) have become steadily less happy, more insecure, more depressed, and more suicidal (Twenge et al. 2018). In general, there is evidence that these habit-forming technologies decrease our sense of closeness, connectedness, and ability to focus and enjoy life (Dwyer et al. 2018; Hughes and Burke 2018), but the case is far from proven. Social media and the internet may or may not make us more stressed and less happy. Even if they do, they may or may not contribute to mental illness. We simply do not yet know how to understand the pervasive effects of technology on our nervous systems.

One thing does seem likely: Mental illness is common, and it will not decline in the near future. The COVID-19 pandemic has brought a period of major stress, disruption, and uncertainty to the lives of virtually everyone on the planet. Massive unemployment, financial problems, and social isolation only raise the risk that more people will develop mental illness. Adults report experiencing more anxiety and depression (Vindegaard and Benros 2020), and children are at higher risk of educational problems and maltreatment (Fegert et al. 2020). The effects of the pandemic on our mental health are likely to last for many years, perhaps for generations. So mental illness is not going anywhere, and it will continue to affect us all.

How Could These Numbers Be So Large?

Another common reaction to these colossal numbers is to doubt that they could be true. Is it really possible that half of all people experience some kind of mental health problem in life, and one fourth in each year? I do not blame anyone for being skeptical about these data. I myself was skeptical for many years. When these very large studies began to come out in the 1990s, I had deep doubts about them. I knew I was biased—unlike most people, I was a psychiatrist and someone who had experienced mental illness. I saw mental illness and thought about mental illness all day pretty much every day. I knew I might be off base, but had guessed that up to 20% or so of the population might experience mental illness in the lifetime. As these studies came out, the results were so much larger than I expected that I did not completely trust them for years. It took many studies and a lot of background research to feel any degree of confidence about them.

So maybe these studies are badly overestimating mental illness. Maybe we have one of those situations in which the more we look, the more we are going to find. Keep asking people if they have had mental illness, and eventually they will say yes. Keep telling people that mental illness is common, and maybe they will just assume they have had it. Maybe we are all convincing each other of its reality, like people in the 1950s used to fear that communists were everywhere undermining society. Then again, maybe recent generations have had it too easy. Perhaps we are not as tough as previous generations, so we assume that we have some kind of a disorder when really life is just difficult, painful, and exhausting.

These things are possible, of course. We should take such questions seriously. We do not do any favors for people with true mental illness if we trivialize the whole idea of having mental illness. We should not call all sadness depression, or all worry anxiety. Everyone has stress (as we shall discuss in Chapter 7), but stress is not an illness. If we regard normal life pains and stresses as illnesses, we cast doubt on those who are diagnosed with real illnesses. We should not call people with normal stress medically ill, and we certainly should not prescribe psychiatric medications or other treatments to people who do not truly have an illness. Medications treat diseases, not problems, as one of my teachers used to say. Overdiagnosis and overtreatment can do serious harm to innocent people, so we should not be too quick to say that people have mental illness. Instead, let's take a deeper look at just how solid these numbers might be.

First, the size of the numbers is astounding, but should that alone make us doubtful? Is it possible that 50% of the population can have one kind of medical illness? In fact, there are many medical illnesses that are exceedingly common (Figure 3–2). For instance, 90% of the U.S. population will develop high blood pressure (hypertension) at some point in life. Most of these cases are mild, but 40% of us will still experience moderate to severe high blood pressure (Vasan et al. 2002). Forty percent of Americans will experience cancer at some time in life (Howlader et al. 2020). And the lifetime risk of heart disease is about 50% for men and 40% for women (Lloyd-Jones et al. 2006). In this context, the lifetime risk of mental illness does not seem to be out of proportion; mental illness is about as common as many other chronic diseases.

If we look more deeply, we can also evaluate the quality of the studies that gave us these numbers. One thing to notice is that they are large surveys—very large. All of them involve many thousands of people—8,000 to 50,000, to be precise. By comparison, the traditional number for a Gallup-type poll is about 1,000 people, a number that is regarded as large enough for an accurate national survey, if the survey is well done. Of course, numbers alone are not enough. The people surveyed have to be representative of the country as a whole. And like other well-done surveys, the people in these studies accurately represented our national ethnic and cultural diversity.

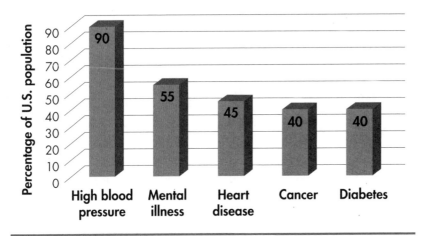

FIGURE 3–2. Lifetime risk[a] of common chronic illnesses.

[a]Percentage of the population developing the disease during their lifetime.
Source. Adapted from Gregg et al. 2014; Howlader et al. 2020; Kessler et al. 2007; Lloyd-Jones et al. 2006; Vasan et al. 2002.

Furthermore, the researchers did not simply call these people on the phone and say, "Hi, we're doing a survey on mental illness today. Do you have mental illness? Yes or no? Great—thanks for your answer!" and hang up. The surveys involved in-person meetings. The questions were detailed, comprehensive, and specific. For instance, the federal government's National Survey on Drug Use and Health (NSDUH) takes about an hour to complete (Substance Abuse and Mental Health Services Administration 2018b). The evaluation for the landmark National Comorbidity Survey Replication (NCS-R) took 45 minutes to 2 hours (World Health Organization World Mental Health Composite International Diagnostic Interview 2020). These surveys have been developed and tested over decades so that they will be both consistent (reliable) and accurate (valid) in their results. No test involving human beings is perfect, and different studies have used different tests, and this makes for some differences in the results. But compared to most other survey data we hear about, we can have a high degree of confidence in these measurements (Hedden et al. 2012; see also Kessler et al. 2005a).

Finally, looking more deeply shows us that results between studies are consistent: Independent national studies have generally produced results that agree with each other. These results also fit with data from many smaller studies. So the numbers about mental illness hardly represent a "flash in the pan." They are based on many studies, and many years of work. The research is so extensive that there are no serious scientific challenges to the surveys. There are no researchers asserting that the studies are invalid because they are poorly done, or that better surveys would show vastly different results. Even worldwide, where such studies are often more difficult to undertake, the results are generally consistent (Kessler et al. 2007).

How Do We Know We Are Measuring Something Real?

Although there is no debate about the quality of the studies involved, there are people with deeper doubts about the results of these studies. I do not blame them for being skeptical. These people wonder what the studies are measuring in the first place. Are studies measuring only mental illness, or do they also include people with normal stresses? Even mental health professionals can cringe at the size of the results. Could there really be such an "epidemic" of mental illness? Look around you. Do you see mental illness everywhere? These claims are enormous and seem to go against common sense. It is hard for most people to believe that so many could be medically ill with this one type of medical problem. As one mental health advocate put it, "Psychiatry groups represent...[an] extreme: They believe almost everything is a mental illness. Their literature claims up to 50% of people had a 'diagnosable' mental disorder during their life.... They believe that almost every feeling...and social issue...are mental illnesses that need earlier and earlier identification, treatment and often an expensive new medication" (Jaffe 2020).

So, even if we are doing a good job of measuring rates of mental disorders, there is a further question: What are we measuring? Are we just calling everything mental illness? Do these numbers reflect true medical illnesses or just normal human problems and feelings? Maybe *depression* is just another word for sadness, and *schizophrenia* is just another way of labeling the eccentric. In other words, psychiatrists and other researchers could be defining and measuring something that is not even an illness at all. Mental illness could be a made-up set of labels, or it could be something medical and real. But which is it? Could mental illness turn out to be a myth, or is it truly real?

Advice for Advocacy

- You can walk into any and every room confident that everyone in that room is personally affected by mental illness. Remind yourself that this information is relevant and important to everyone.

- Many people will not know that they are affected. They will forget about their own young adult substance problems, their spouse's depression, or their childhood friend with severe mental illness. But you can remind them. And you can confidently assure them that they are personally connected to those with mental illness, whether or not they know it.

- Remember that many people you address do know that they and people they love have had mental illness. These individuals will be relieved by the evidence that they are neither deviant nor outliers.

- Some will respond to this information with enthusiasm. Others will seem wary and guarded. Remember that a sense of tension or resistance is also a sign that people are engaging. If they are having doubts about the realities of mental illness, you know you have their attention and the ability to address those doubts.

- It often helps to admit that these numbers are huge, much higher than most people would reasonably expect. You can then go on to explain how much research and validation is behind them. This helps you identify with "doubters" but go on to show that the data are well substantiated even if counterintuitive.

- Graphs and verbal illustrations will have more emotional impact than numbers alone. People need to hear the numbers, but then they need the illustrations to help them visualize the meaning and importance of those numbers. Give them the data in a brief and concise way, then go on to talk relatably about the significance of the data.

References

Centers for Disease Control and Prevention: Key facts about influenza (flu). September 13, 2019. Available at: www.cdc.gov/flu/about/keyfacts.htm. Accessed July 23, 2020.

Dittman M: Hughes's germ phobia revealed in psychological autopsy. Monitor on Psychology 36(7):102, 2005

Dwyer RJ, Kushlev K, Dunn EW: Smartphone use undermines enjoyment of face-to-face social interactions. J Exp Soc Psychol 78:233–239, 2018

Fegert JM, Vitiello B, Plener PL, Clemens V: Challenges and burden of the Coronavirus 2019 (COVID-19) pandemic for child and adolescent mental health: a narrative review to highlight clinical and research needs in the acute phase and the long return to normality. Child Adolesc Psychiatry Ment Health 14:20, 2020

Greenwald AG: The totalitarian ego: fabrication and revision of personal history. Am Psychol 35(7):603–618, 1980

Gregg EW, Zhuo X, Cheng YJ, et al: Trends in lifetime risk and years of life lost due to diabetes in the USA, 1985–2011: a modelling study. Lancet Diabetes Endocrinol 2(11):867–874, 2014

Hasin DS, Grant BF: The National Epidemiologic Survey on Alcohol and Related Conditions (NESARC) Waves 1 and 2: review and summary of findings. Soc Psychiatry Psychiatr Epidemiol 50(11):1609–1640, 2015

Hedden S, Gfroerer J, Barker P, et al: Comparison of NSDUH mental health data and methods with other data sources. CBHSQ Data Review, February 2012. Available at: www.ncbi.nlm.nih.gov/books/NBK390286/pdf/Bookshelf_NBK390286.pdf. Accessed July 23, 2020.

Hidaka BH: Depression as a disease of modernity: explanations for increasing prevalence. J Affect Disord 140(3):205–214, 2012

Howlader N, Noone AM, Krapcho M, et al (eds): SEER Cancer Statistics Review, 1975–2016. National Cancer Institute, April 9, 2020. Available at: https://seer.cancer.gov/csr/1975_2016. Accessed July 23, 2020.

Hughes N, Burke J: Sleeping with the frenemy: how restricting "bedroom use" of smartphones impacts happiness and wellbeing. Comput Human Behav 85:236–244, 2018

Jaffe DJ: Antipsychiatry vs. psychiatry. Mental Illness Policy Org, 2020. Available at: https://mentalillnesspolicy.org/myths/antipsychiatry.html. Accessed July 23, 2020.

Jamison KR: Touched With Fire. New York, Simon & Schuster, 1996

Kaiser Permanente: Highlights from a new national consumer poll. Find Your Words, 2018. Available at: https://findyourwords.org/mental-health-myths-facts-national-poll. Accessed July 23, 2020.

Kennedy PJ, Fried S: A Common Struggle: A Personal Journey Through the Past and Future of Mental Illness and Addiction. New York, Penguin, 2016

Kessler RC, McGonagle KA, Zhao S, et al: Lifetime and 12-month prevalence of DSM-III-R psychiatric disorders in the United States: results from the National Comorbidity Survey. Arch Gen Psychiatry 51(1):8–19, 1994

Kessler RC, Anthony JC, Blazer DG, et al: The US National Comorbidity Survey: overview and future directions. Epidemiol Psychiatr Soc 6(1):4–16, 1997

Kessler RC, Berglund P, Demler O, et al: Lifetime prevalence and age-of-onset distributions of DSM-IV disorders in the National Comorbidity Survey Replication. Arch Gen Psychiatry 62(6):593–602, 2005a

Kessler RC, Chiu WT, Demler O, et al: Prevalence, severity, and comorbidity of 12-month DSM-IV disorders in the National Comorbidity Survey Replication. Arch Gen Psychiatry 62(6):617–627, 2005b

Kessler RC, Angermeyer M, Anthony JC, et al: Lifetime prevalence and age-of-onset distributions of mental disorders in the World Health Organization's World Mental Health Survey Initiative. World Psychiatry 6(3):168–176, 2007

Keyes CL: Promoting and protecting mental health as flourishing: a complementary strategy for improving national mental health. Am Psychol 62(2):95–108, 2007

Leary MR: Self-Presentation: Impression Management and Interpersonal Behavior. New York, Routledge, 2019

Lloyd-Jones DM, Leip EP, Larson MG, et al: Prediction of lifetime risk for cardiovascular disease by risk factor burden at 50 years of age. Circulation 113(6):791–798, 2006

Matson JL, Kozlowski AM: The increasing prevalence of autism spectrum disorders. Res Autism Spectr Disord 5(1):418–425, 2011

Omran AR: The epidemiologic transition: a theory of the epidemiology of population change. Milbank Mem Fund Q 49(4):509–538, 1971

Parcesepe AM, Cabassa LJ: Public stigma of mental illness in the United States: a systematic literature review. Adm Policy Ment Health 40(5):384–399, 2013

Perälä J, Suvisaari J, Saarni SI, et al: Lifetime prevalence of psychotic and bipolar I disorders in a general population. Arch Gen Psychiatry 64(1):19–28, 2007

Pies R: Bogus "epidemic" of mental illness in the US. Psychiatric Times, June 18, 2015. Available at: www.psychiatrictimes.com/blogs/bogus-epidemic-mental-illness-us. Accessed July 23, 2020.

Pinker S: The Better Angels of Our Nature: Why Violence Has Declined. New York, Penguin, 2012

Regier DA, Myers JK, Kramer M, et al: The NIMH Epidemiologic Catchment Area program: historical context, major objectives, and study population characteristics. Arch Gen Psychiatry 41(10):934–941, 1984

Shenk JW: Lincoln's Melancholy: How Depression Challenged a President and Fueled His Greatness. New York, Houghton Mifflin Harcourt, 2006

Substance Abuse and Mental Health Services Administration: Key Substance Use and Mental Health Indicators in the United States: Results From the 2017 National Survey on Drug Use and Health (HHS Publ No SMA 18-5068, NSDUH Series H-53). 2018a. Available at: www.samhsa.gov/data/sites/default/files/cbhsq-reports/NSDUHFFR2017/NSDUHFFR2017.pdf. Accessed July 23, 2020.

Substance Abuse and Mental Health Services Administration: 2019 National Survey on Drug Use and Health (NSDUH): Final CAI Specifications for Programming (English version). October 18, 2018b. Available at: www.samhsa.gov/data/sites/default/files/cbhsq-reports/NSDUHmrbCAISpecs2019.pdf. Accessed July 23, 2020.

Twenge JM, Joiner TE, Rogers ML, et al: Increases in depressive symptoms, suicide-related outcomes, and suicide rates among US adolescents after 2010 and links to increased new media screen time. Clin Psychol Sci 6(1):3–17, 2018

U.S. Census Bureau: Quick facts, persons under 5 years, percent. 2020. Available at: www.census.gov/quickfacts/fact/table/US/AGE135219. Accessed July 23, 2020.

Vasan RS, Beiser A, Seshadri S, et al: Residual lifetime risk for developing hypertension in middle-aged women and men: the Framingham Heart Study. JAMA 287(8):1003–1010, 2002

Vindegaard N, Benros ME: COVID-19 pandemic and mental health consequences: systematic review of the current evidence. Brain Behav Immun 89:531–542, 2020

World Health Organization World Mental Health Composite International Diagnostic Interview (WHO WMH-CIDI): About the WHO WMH-CIDI: New Sampling Conventions for the Paper and Pencil Version (PAPI). 2020. Available at: www.hcp.med.harvard.edu/wmhcidi/about-the-who-wmh-cidi/#jump2_d. Accessed July 23, 2020.

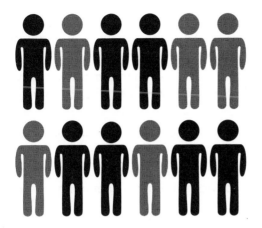

Is Mental Illness a Myth?

Half Truth: Some people think mental health diagnosis and treatment is a fraud, whereas other people think it is a medical necessity.

Whole Truth: All of us who care about mental illness are trying to figure out what people with mental illness really have and what they really need.

Important Points

- In 1961, Dr. Thomas Szasz wrote *The Myth of Mental Illness*, an influential book arguing that mental illness is not real medical illness.
- Many serious people today, including some psychiatrists, psychologists, journalists, and professors, doubt that mental illness is true medical illness.

- They argue that psychiatrists overdiagnose and overprescribe medications for illnesses that may not even be illnesses.
- Millions of people are getting mental health treatment right now, yet millions more who have mental illness are not getting treatment for it.
- This great cultural debate leaves people hesitant and uncertain about whether or not to get treatment.
- We need to take these concerns seriously, look carefully at whether mental illness is real, and decide whether it should be treated like other medical illnesses.

Introduction

If "mental illness is common" represents the best-supported statement in psychiatry, then "psychiatrists are making up mental illness" represents the deepest criticism. This latter statement rests on an understandable misunderstanding of DSM—that is, on the partial truth that committees composed primarily of psychiatrists get together and vote on what constitutes mental illness. The second most important criticism about mental health practice is that psychiatrists (and others) overprescribe medications for their own profit. These two criticisms—overdiagnosis and overprescription—paint a picture of mental health professionals as unscientific, self-deceptive, self-interested, and greedy.

I think that these criticisms should be acknowledged and named, but I do not believe that advocacy is a proper setting for debating them in detail. We as advocates do not need to focus either on the details of DSM or on a discussion of whether psychiatry is a self-serving "industry." These questions are important but belong to other types of forums. Instead, we can take these criticisms as welcome intellectual challenges to more important and fundamental questions: Is there really such a thing as mental illness? Is mental illness medically real? Do medications really help people who have mental illness? These are the questions we want people to care about, and the criticisms bring a sense of emotional urgency and interest that these questions deserve. Antipsychiatry critiques bring a sense of heightened drama that truly belongs to these discussions. The nature of mental illness and its treatment is of overwhelming importance, and critics of psychiatry do give it such importance. But we will not answer the relevant questions through long examinations of DSM and its formation. Instead, we can together look more deeply into the scientific foundations of mental health care, a vast web of research that can tell us definitively about the nature of mental illness and its treatment.

In this sense, we should invite everyone to the discussion: People who criticize psychiatry presumably want the same thing as people who are treating mental illness. All of us want to help those who are troubled, who deal with psychosis, suicidality, depression, overwhelming anger, trauma, and addiction. All of us want to understand what is best for such problems. All of us are interested in the truth. Therefore, advocacy does not involve rejecting our critics, but rather inviting them to examine the scientific evidence for the foundations of mental health care.

Who Would Doubt a Psychiatrist?

I am a psychiatrist, but I have to say it: Most people are not too sure about psychiatrists. When I meet new people, things are friendly until they ask what I do. "I am a psychiatrist." "Oh! Well," comes the most common answer, "you could sure make a career off me (or my family, or this town, etc.)." We both laugh, and then there are no more comments about my being a psychiatrist. Often people are wary for a while after that, as if I am secretly analyzing them. I do understand that most people hope they never have to see a psychiatrist. No one should want mental illness any more than another any other illness, and no one should want to see a psychiatrist any more than any other kind of doctor. At the same it, the wariness goes way beyond medical illness and treatment. Both psychiatrists and psychologists, after all, are commonly known as "shrinks." *Shrink* is short for "head shrinker," apparently referring to an Amazon tribe that literally shrank the heads of enemies after death. The term also seems to be related to *witch doctor*, another term for psychiatrists. This idea implies that (unlike other doctors) psychiatrists use superstition, magic, fear, and mystery. They are both scary and laughable, practicing something that might be dangerous and fake at the same time. Whatever it is they do, it is not straightforward medicine. Witch doctors are different from medical doctors, and psychiatrists have often been more like witch doctors than medical doctors in the public's imagination.

To this day, there are large groups of people who doubt the whole idea of psychiatry as medical practice. Some of these skeptics even include psychiatrists. Part of the criticism is that psychiatrists are pill pushers, or even drug dealers. But there is a more basic criticism, one that concerns the very existence of mental illness. It is well summarized by Gumba Gumba, a contributor to the online *Urban Dictionary*, who defined a shrink as "someone who matches your symptoms to whatever random disorder they've just pulled out of their ass" (Urban Dictionary 2004). In other words, a psychiatrist is someone who makes up mental illnesses. And Gumba Gumba is not the only one who thinks so. There are many serious critics of mental health care who say the same. They include college professors, writers, and cultural critics, and notably psychiatrists and psychologists. They are serious, educated people who disagree that mental illness is medical. They present a very different picture of mental illness: They claim that mental illness is cultural and not biological—that mental illness is whatever the culture defines as "insane" or deviant rather than being the result of some objective biological dysfunction. Why do they say so?

Mental Illness: Fact or Fiction?

In 1961, Dr. Thomas Szasz published *The Myth of Mental Illness*. The book quickly became a classic and remains deeply influential to this day. It remains in print with a fiftieth anniversary edition, and is still quoted with approval in numerous books, articles, and blogs (Kelly et al. 2010). Szasz was a powerful writer who drove home the core idea of the book from its very first words. No one who reads even the title of his book will ever forget it.

Thomas Szasz was a medical doctor and psychiatrist. But he thought there was a deep difference between the two. He did not think that being a medical doctor had much to do with being a psychiatrist. In fact, he thought that calling psychiatry a branch of medicine was a terrible idea, fundamentally wrong and destructive. He practiced psychiatry as a psychotherapist, but he did not prescribe medicines or claim that he was acting as a medical doctor. Instead, he claimed he was helping people deal with life problems, which he said were not medical but moral.

Szasz went straight to the heart of the matter, which is why his book is still cited on a regular basis. He flatly stated that mental illness is not biological illness. He said that all illness, by definition, is biological dysfunction. For illness to exist, the body must be unable to function properly. But mental illness, he said, is mental. No one can show that it is biological, and so mental illness is a contradiction in terms. If it is mental, it cannot be physical. Accordingly, no one could show Szasz that it is physical.

"Psychiatry is traditionally defined as a medical specialty concerned with the diagnosis and treatment of mental diseases. I submit that this definition, which is still widely accepted, places psychiatry in the company of alchemy and astrology and commits it to the category of pseudoscience. The reason is that there is no such thing as 'mental illness'" (Szasz 1961, p. 1).

Those were the first three sentences of the whole book, but they summarized the rest of it quite powerfully.

Szasz said that calling in a medical doctor to treat mental illness would be like calling a television repair technician to fix a bad TV program. What he meant was that a physically ill body is like a broken television set—in either case, one should call in a technician to fix the "hardware." On the other hand, mental problems are like the television program itself and cannot be fixed by tinkering with the hardware. Szasz was clear that medical illness refers to a "physiochemical abnormality" (Szasz 1961, p. 83), a biological defect of some kind. He differentiated this from a "psychosocial communication" (Szasz 1961, p. 84), a problem with the software and not the hardware. He thought that a few mental problems are due to medical illnesses such as brain tumors, but that everything else labeled "mental illness" is merely a deviation from social and ethical norms (Szasz 1960).

Dr. Szasz thought that calling people mentally ill was not doing them any favors. Rather, it encouraged them to see themselves as sick and unable to function. It asked them to passively wait for the doctor's diagnosis, then passively take whatever medicine or other treatment the doctor recommended. He insisted the label of mental illness took away power and responsibility from so-called patients. Rejecting this "medical metaphor," Szasz believed in telling people that they could be responsible for their own problems and in helping them take control of their lives.

No one should oppose the effort to empower people with respect to their own lives and problems. But Thomas Szasz argued that doctors did just that by pretending to treat "mental illness." This illusion of medical treatment could only get in the way of people being responsible and empowered, limiting their sense of freedom and choice. It weakened them rather than strengthened them, plaguing them with unnecessary and even dangerous "treatments" in the process. Therefore (said Szasz) medical psychiatry was blatantly wrong and grossly unethical at the same time. Licensed as a medical doctor, Szasz refused to practice medicine and instead offered only counseling. "I am probably the only psychiatrist in the world whose hands are clean," he told a reporter after his retirement. "I have never committed anyone. I have never given electric shock. I have never, ever given drugs to a mental patient" (Maugh 2012).

The Myth of the Myth of Mental Illness

What are we to make of this powerful work today? In my opinion, we need to remember two things about *The Myth of Mental Illness*. First, when he wrote the book in the late 1950s, Szasz was essentially right. No one could show him that mental illness was physical dysfunction. No one could take the brain of someone with schizophrenia or any other mental illness and show that there was something physically wrong with that brain. In the vast majority of cases, there was no reason to believe that mental illness was physical, and every reason to believe that it was mental. So Szasz was right, at the time he wrote his book.

The second thing we should remember about *The Myth of Mental Illness* is that it was written in the late 1950s, and the 1950s were a long time ago. Szasz started writing his book in 1954 (Szasz 1961, p. vii), which also happened to be the last year that a medical doctor endorsed cigarettes in an ad campaign (Gardner and Brandt 2006). In that era, racial segregation was the norm, and a "woman's place was in the home." Our culture has changed profoundly since that time, and so has science. A scientific revolution has transformed the field of neuroscience (brain science). When Szasz wrote his book, there were no head scanning technologies, such as computed tomography (CT) and magnetic resonance imaging (MRI); no information about neurotransmitters (such as serotonin and dopamine); and few psychiatric medications. Thorazine, the first psychiatric medication to be widely used, had just been recognized in 1953, and antidepressants only emerged in the late 1950s. The average stay in a state mental hospital in 1950 was 11 years (Kramer 2005), mostly because there were few effective treatments. If we exclude alcohol (a popular unofficial psychiatric medication of the time), then talk therapy was the main treatment available. And there were no scientific studies proving that even talk therapy was effective for mental illness.

Ironically, the neuroscience revolution was just starting in the 1950s (Shepherd 2009), although its effects would not be felt until years later. To be fair to Szasz, he held on tenaciously to his opinions about psychiatry for the rest of his life, which ended in 2012 at the age of 92. Four years before, he had cleared up any remaining uncertainty about his views by publishing *Psychiatry: The Science of Lies* (Szasz 2008). Notably, Szasz has not been alone in his tenacious criticism of mental illness and psychiatry. A large number of people still agree with Szasz. Critics with similar opinions have detailed and updated these ideas with *New York Times* best sellers (Hari 2018; Whitaker 2010), articles in academic journals (Pilgrim 2007), various books by famous authors (Figure 4–1), countless websites (e.g., Keirsey 2011), and books by a host of psychiatrists and psychotherapists (e.g., Breggin 1994; Greenberg 2014). One psychologist wrote the following:

> Tom Szasz was the clearest thinker and writer that I have known; his influence has been to help me see and think more clearly, especially in regard to my work. It began with *The Myth of Mental Illness*; despite the ongoing mas-

sive denial of the undeniable—that the concept of mental illness is a metaphor, and that psychiatry failed 52 years ago, and still fails, to meet the… standard of disease as a confirmable physical or chemical abnormality in regard to the myriad 'mental illnesses' extant today—I have remained able to see the distinction between a metaphor and an objective disease. (Breeding 2014)

Although I am going to show that scientific progress has definitively answered Szasz's challenge to the "myth" of mental illness, the debate is not over (Phillips et al. 2012). There are still university professors, prominent journalists, powerful nonprofit corporations, boards of experts (Cooke 2014), and at times even government agencies (McCance-Katz 2016; Torrey 2014) that support the idea that mental illness should not be treated as medical illness. So before making a scientific response to *The Myth of Mental Illness*, let me summarize the current opinions of these critics of mental illness.

The Myth of Mental Illness Today

Present-day critics of mental illness generally focus on the work of psychiatrists. In one way, this makes sense: Psychiatrists are the medical specialists who treat mental illness. Psychiatrists are the main group that defines mental illness and its treatment. On the other hand, mental health treatment has always been a team effort (Menninger 1998). Psychologists, social workers, nurses, nurse practitioners, and physician's assistants are all vitally involved in mental health treatment. They are all trained professionals who have complementary roles in our health care system. Families too are a major part of treatment and usually have a large role to play. And no treatment for mental illness ultimately succeeds without the patient, the person dealing with the mental illness. That person is the most important part of the treatment team.

You might think that there is one exception to this team approach—it's the psychiatrists who prescribe the medications, after all. But even prescribing is a team effort. Psychiatrists depend on nonprescribers (such as nurses, psychologists, social workers, family members, and most of all patients) to give feedback on whether medicines are helping or hurting, and what symptoms need to be treated. Patients ultimately make the decision of whether to take a medicine, not doctors. In addition, nurse practitioners, physician's assistants, and (in some states) psychologists prescribe. Most people do not realize that *psychiatrists do not prescribe most of the psychiatric medications in this*

We've Had a Hundred Years of Psychotherapy—and the World's Getting Worse (Hillman and Ventura 1992)

Toxic Psychiatry: Why Therapy, Empathy, and Love Must Replace the Drugs, Electroshock, and Biochemical Theories of the "New Psychiatry" (Breggin 1994)

Your Drug May Be Your Problem: How and Why to Stop Taking Psychiatric Medications (Breggin and Cohen 1999)

Mad in America: Bad Science, Bad Medicine, and the Enduring Mistreatment of the Mentally Ill (Whitaker 2002)

Warning: Psychiatry Can Be Hazardous to Your Mental Health (Glasser 2003)

The Great Psychiatry Scam: One Shrink's Personal Journey (Ross 2008)

Unhinged: The Trouble With Psychiatry—A Doctor's Revelations About a Profession in Crisis (Carlat 2010)

Anatomy of an Epidemic: Magic Bullets, Psychiatric Drugs, and the Astonishing Rise of Mental Illness in America (Whitaker 2010)

Pharmageddon (Healy 2012)

The Loss of Sadness: How Psychiatry Transformed Normal Sorrow Into Depressive Disorder (Horwitz and Wakefield 2012)

Cracked: Why Psychiatry Is Doing More Harm Than Good (Davies 2014)

Saving Normal: An Insider's Revolt Against Out-of-Control Psychiatric Diagnosis, DSM-5, Big Pharma, and the Medicalization of Ordinary Life (Frances 2013)

Book of Woe: The DSM and the Unmaking of Psychiatry (Greenberg 2014)

Psychiatry Under the Influence: Institutional Corruption, Social Injury, and Prescriptions for Reform (Whitaker and Cosgrove 2015)

ADHD Nation: Children, Doctors, Big Pharma, and the Making of an American Epidemic (Schwarz 2016)

Lost Connections: Uncovering the Real Causes of Depression—and the Unexpected Solutions (Hari 2018)

Anxiety—The Inside Story: How Biological Psychiatry Got It Wrong (McLaren 2018)

Mind Fixers: Psychiatry's Troubled Search for the Biology of Mental Illness (Harrington 2019)

FIGURE 4–1. Books critical of mental health diagnosis and care: a selection.

country. Primary care doctors (such as family physicians) prescribe most of them. In fact, primary care doctors prescribe 59% of all psychiatric medications (Mark et al. 2009). So it is not just psychiatrists who are the heroes or villains here. It is the whole medical system. Governments, insurance companies, universities, and hospitals all have a big influence in how the system works. That being said, I will use the term *psychiatrists* to refer to all mental health and medical treaters who address mental illness. And I will use *psychiatry* to indicate that we are talking about the medical treatment of mental illness, the view that mental illness is a real medical problem.

The most common criticism of psychiatry today is detailed in countless books and goes as follows: Psychiatrists are too eager to prescribe medicines. They are too eager to prescribe medicines because it is good for business—psychiatrists make money from seeing patients and prescribing medicines, and drug companies make money by convincing psychiatrists to prescribe more medicines. Both psychiatrists and drug companies want to classify more and more people as mentally ill, because then more people will need more medications. So psychiatrists (with the help of drug companies) define more and more people as mentally ill. How do they do this? By finding new "mental illnesses," but even more by broadening the definitions of old mental illnesses. How can they pull this off? By getting together in committees and taking votes on what defines a mental illness. How can psychiatrists just take a vote and change the definitions to include more people? Because psychiatry is not really based on science, but rather is based on a culture masquerading as science. Mental illness is a myth. There is no bedrock scientific foundation for psychiatry as there is for other branches of medicine. This lack of a solid foundation means that the whole practice of psychiatry can be corrupted by financial and other interests.

Ultimately, the argument rests on whether psychiatry has a scientific basis. That is the most fundamental question about the nature and treatment of mental illness: Is it based on medical science in the same way that other medical specialties are? But the critics' argument is complicated, so let's break it down into its separate layers:

1. Psychiatry is not based on hard biological science. Psychiatry is not like other branches of medicine. It is not about bodily dysfunction that requires biological treatment; it is about "mental illnesses," which we do not really understand.
2. Because psychiatry is not based on hard science, it is based on the opinions of psychiatrists. If we say that psychiatry is based on the *opinions* of a group of people (psychiatrists), then we are saying that mental illness is a matter of social or cultural definition. In other words, "mental illness" is an idea that can be very different in some cultures and may not exist at all in

others. Mental illness can be defined in pretty much any way a group defines it. Mental illness is a cultural construct, not a physical reality.

3. Psychiatrists get to define mental illness. They are the so-called experts on mental illness in our society. So they define mental illness in the way that suits psychiatrists. What do psychiatrists want? Psychiatrists want to have the authority of medical doctors, so they claim psychiatry is a medical science. And they want power over people, so they claim that more and more people are mentally ill.

4. How do psychiatrists change the definitions of mental illnesses? They get together in committees and make formal definitions of mental illnesses. They decide when to diagnose a person with major depression or schizophrenia by making up a list of symptoms. These definitions are enshrined in DSM (now in its fifth edition, DSM-5; American Psychiatric Association 2013), and medical professionals everywhere follow DSM to diagnose people. So do insurance companies. So do Medicare and Medicaid. Because they can define mental illnesses any way they wish, psychiatrists make the definitions more and more broad. As a result, people who used to be classified as normal become classified as mentally ill.

5. When more people are classified as mentally ill, more people need more psychiatrists and more medicines. This is good for the business of psychiatry, and good for drug companies that sell the medications. Psychiatrists do not really want people to get other kinds of relief from mental symptoms, because that would be bad for business. Psychiatrists are the ones who prescribe pills, so they recommend pills over other options such as talk therapy and social support.

6. More and more people wind up taking psychiatric medications and being classified as mentally ill. But since the medicines do more harm than good, most people do not get better. They continue to have problems and try more and more pills rather than other options. Thus, more and more people struggle with "mental illness," and when they do not get better, they go back for more pills. So the problem just continues and expands in a vicious cycle. When the old medicines fail to work, the drug companies just come up with new medicines, and psychiatrists are happy to try them in order to keep people coming back.

Admittedly, all that was a bit complicated. On the other hand, we have just encapsulated quite a few well-known critiques of psychiatry in a few paragraphs (see Figure 4–1). So let's sum it all up: 1) Psychiatry is not based on medical science, so 2) it is based on the opinions of a group of people and therefore is a cultural construct. 3) That group of people comprises psychiatrists, who define mental illnesses in order to call more and more people mentally ill 4) by means of DSM, which they themselves created. 5) This means that more and more people need to go to psychiatrists for treatment, and more and more people get put on psychiatric medications. 6) As these people feel worse rather than better, they return to get put on more psychiatric medications in a vicious and corrupt cycle of victimization.

I hope you can see that the critics have a real case to make. Their arguments make sense, as far as they go. So they need to be addressed. And I hope that something else is also clear: The whole debate comes down to whether psychiatry is based on science or based on something else. That is the most important question to ask about mental illness and its treatment. It is not just an academic debate. It affects the lives of millions of people right now—people who took a psychiatric medication just this morning, people who have been labeled as having mental illness, people who have been in a psychiatric hospital or treatment center, people who are suffering horribly at this moment and needing some relief. It affects people in my family and probably yours. It really matters to all of them even if they do not think about this particular question: Is mental illness and its treatment physically real and based on science?

The Antipsychiatry Debate: Does It Really Matter?

There is one very specific reason to take these arguments seriously: There are practical consequences to our ambivalence about mental health and its treatment. Ironically, the vast majority of Americans endorse the idea that mental illness is legitimate medical illness (Universal Health Services 2019). At the same time, a majority of them (60%) do not receive any treatment when they suffer from mental health disorders (Substance Abuse and Mental Health Services Administration 2018). And even when people do get treatment, half or more do not continue their treatments as prescribed (Dufort and Zipursky 2019; Jawad et al. 2018; Sawada et al. 2009). The vast majority of people with mental illness do not get consistent treatment for it. And so Americans remain of two minds about mental disorders: On the one hand they affirm that mental illnesses are real and treatable, but on the other they usually avoid treatment for them.

On top of this, most people who do seek treatment actually delay doing so for years after the disorder begins. A small minority get treatment within the first year, but on average people have symptoms for over 10 years before seeking treatment (McGorry et al. 2011; Wang et al. 2005). Delays may cause years of additional suffering, and can also worsen the course of illness. If mental illness really is medical, prompt treatment will work better, and the illness usually deepens if left untreated. Therefore, waiting on treatment not only delays relief but also can worsen the illness for the person who has it, as well as worsen their ultimate response to treatment (Dell'Osso et al. 2013). This does not mean that people who wait are doomed, as we will see in Chapter 8. But the stakes of this debate are very high, and literally life-changing.

There are many reasons for these delays—sometimes people cannot find someone to treat them, and sometimes they cannot afford the treatment. Limitations in insurance coverage are a massive problem, even when people have insurance. But surely our cultural uncertainty about mental health treatment is another reason. Studies have shown that people who feel shame and self-negativity about a mental health diagnosis are less likely to stay with treatment (Livingston and Boyd 2010). We have deep cultural doubts about whether we can trust mental health diagnosis and treatment, and those doubts can only feed the uncertainty of people who are on the fence about seeking treatment.

The majority of Americans seem wary of the mental health establishment. The dominant media narrative is that psychiatry is "troubled" and "in crisis," possibly even harmful and corrupt. There is little coverage of successful mental health treatment and recovery (McGinty et al. 2016). Major national news outlets, such as the *The New York Times* (Szalai 2019), *The Atlantic* (Greenberg 2019), and *The New Yorker* (Groopman 2019), periodically publish reviews critical of mental health treatment. They routinely report that psychiatry lacks a scientific basis, that people are vastly overtreated, and that misguided diagnosis and treatment efforts are reckless and harmful. If people are repeatedly told that they are overdiagnosed and overmedicated, then some are likely to hesitate to the point of desperation before seeking help. Although most people say that mental illness is real (see Chapter 5), most people do not seem to treat it as real. They do not act as though they believe that mental illness is medical illness with medical treatments. And so they do not pursue treatment.

The question about the nature of mental illness has real-world consequences: On the one hand, if mental illness is a myth, then millions of people are being subjected to medical treatments that can only harm them. On the other hand, if mental illness is medical illness, then our uncertainty is preventing millions of people from getting effective treatment for it. Either way, people will live and die based on our answer to this question. People will die from unnecessary and expensive medical treatments, or people will die from suicide and other consequences of mental illness. We have every reason to make up our minds about this issue, if there is a way to do so. The uncertainty is killing us—literally.

Antipsychiatry: Good or Bad?

I am not personally bothered by these critiques of psychiatry. True, there is an antipsychiatry movement (or more precisely movements; Rissmiller and Rissmiller 2006), while we do not see an anti-nephrology movement or an anti-oncology movement. But differing approaches exist because no one person or group has all the answers about mental health. We are still coming to understand the human brain, and we are still learning how to meet the needs of people with mental illness. We need to bring differing perspectives together in order to address those needs. And the needs are so great that we desperately need to figure out the answers as soon as we possibly can. As both "sides" of the debate agree, people's lives hang in the balance, and not just hundreds and thousands of lives. Millions of people are affected by all of this.

On a deeper level, I am grateful for the critics of psychiatry, and thank them for their work. They care, and they should care. They see problems in our system, and they want to address those problems. They say that this is a matter of life and death, and they are right. We should all be carefully concerned and understand that we are all affected by how we respond to these questions. Happily, the general public does seem interested in mental health, with quite a few major books on psychiatric care published since the turn of the millennium (Figure 4–1). So it is encouraging for me to think that mental health and mental health treatments are so important in our society.

We should also remember than many critics of psychiatry are people who have had negative or wounding experiences in their mental health treatment. Not only do we owe those people a debt to do better, but we should thank them for using their own negative experiences to try and make the system better. We are all in this situation together, though it may not seem like it at times. People with mental health conditions, their families, and mental health professionals all need each other to make progress. And this history of progress (which I will illustrate in this book) is due just as much to people with mental illness and their families as to researchers and medical professionals. We all owe organizations such as NAMI (National Alliance on Mental Illness) a great debt, just as we owe a debt to all the people before us who have tried to understand and overcome mental illness. Finally, we owe a debt to all the people who have challenged our medical system to do better for those with mental illnesses.

In this chapter, I have painted critics of psychiatry with a very broad brush, implying that they all say the same thing. Obviously, this is not the case. There are some on the more extreme end of the spectrum who seem to believe that the world would be better off without any psychiatry at all, and that mental illness itself is a made-up idea (Szasz 1961). There are some who seem to believe that we need mental health treatment, but not with medication or other biological treatments (such as electroconvulsive therapy) (Breggin 1994). Finally, there are some who believe that mental illnesses are real and sometimes need medications, but that psychiatrists have gone overboard in the direction of diagnosing and prescribing (Frances 2013; Schwarz 2016); these critics believe that the problem is with balancing the biological and nonbiological sides of mental illness.

Nevertheless, the criticisms generally point in the same direction: They imply that psychiatry is on the wrong track because it is not carefully limited or firmly based in science. Mental illness is not real because it is not based in science. The diagnosis of mental illness is misguided because it is not based on science. And the treatment of mental illness is out of control because it is not based on science. So let's move forward and address the big question: Is mental illness and its treatment based on science, or not?

Advice for Advocacy

- Most people can readily relate to Szasz's critique of mental illness, even if they do not entirely believe it. They are likely to find his work engaging and stimulating. Discussing his challenges to mental health care puts a human face on the argument, which might otherwise be abstract. And since Szasz was a physician and psychiatrist, you are not demeaning or alienating your audience if you disagree with him.

- Referencing antipsychiatry critiques in your remarks shows that you empathize with differing perspectives, and dealing with them in a nonpolemical way shows that you have more interest in truth than in being proven right. It also helps your listeners, since conscious or unconscious doubts about the reality of mental illness are commonplace.

- Noting these critiques brings a sense of narrative drama to the data you are presenting: Yes, mental illness is common, but some people deny that. They say that mental illness is unreal or made up. They say mental health treatment is overprescribed and even unnecessary. Are they correct? Let's look at the evidence.

- Putting antipsychiatry critiques in a historical context may be the most powerful way of addressing them. At the time they originated (the 1960s and 1970s), they were scientifically legitimate. It is still important to answer these questions. But science has progressed since then, and we now have answers that we lacked in earlier times.

- Remember to stay focused. The nature of DSM is a fascinating and complex topic, as is the question of whether pharmaceutical companies and prescribers promote overprescribing. But these usually distract from the more basic and important questions: Is mental illness medically real? And should mental illness be treated medically (with a biopsychosocial approach)?

- This subtopic is a good chance to make some passing remarks about the astounding progress that has occurred in neuroscience and mental health care since the time of Dr. Szasz's first publications. This information helps inject some positivity and hope into this part of the discussion.

References

American Psychiatric Association: Diagnostic and Statistical Manual of Mental Disorders, 5th Edition. Arlington, VA, American Psychiatric Association, 2013

Breeding J: Practicing Szasz: a psychologist reports on Thomas Szasz's influence on his work. SAGE Open 4(4), 2014

Breggin PR: Toxic Psychiatry: Why Therapy, Empathy, and Love Must Replace the Drugs, Electroshock, and Biochemical Theories of the "New Psychiatry." New York, Macmillan, 1994

Cooke A (ed): Understanding Psychosis and Schizophrenia. British Psychological Society, Division of Clinical Psychology, 2014. www1.bps.org.uk/networks-and-communities/member-microsite/division-clinical-psychology/understanding-psychosis-and-schizophrenia. Accessed July 24, 2020.

Dell'Osso B, Glick ID, Baldwin DS, et al: Can long-term outcomes be improved by shortening the duration of untreated illness in psychiatric disorders? A conceptual framework. Psychopathology 46(1):14–21, 2013

Dufort A, Zipursky RB: Understanding and managing treatment adherence in schizophrenia. Clin Schizophr Relat Psychoses January 3, 2019 [Epub ahead of print]

Frances A: Saving Normal: An Insider's Revolt Against Out-of-Control Psychiatric Diagnosis, DSM-5, Big Pharma, and the Medicalization of Ordinary Life. New York, William Morrow, 2013

Gardner MN, Brandt AM: "The doctors' choice is America's choice": the physician in U.S. cigarette advertisements, 1930–1953. Am J Public Health 96(2):222–232, 2006

Greenberg G: Book of Woe: The DSM and the Unmaking of Psychiatry. New York, Plume, 2014

Greenberg G: Psychiatry's incurable hubris. The Atlantic, April 2019. Available at: www.theatlantic.com/magazine/archive/2019/04/mind-fixers-anne-harrington/583228. Accessed July 24, 2020.

Groopman J: Medicine in mind: psychiatry's fraught history. The New Yorker, May 27, 2019. Available at: www.newyorker.com/magazine/2019/05/27/the-troubled-history-of-psychiatry. Accessed July 24, 2020.

Hari J: Lost Connections: Uncovering the Real Causes of Depression—and the Unexpected Solutions. New York, Bloomsbury, 2018

Jawad I, Watson S, Haddad PM, et al: Medication nonadherence in bipolar disorder: a narrative review. Ther Adv Psychopharmacol 8(12):349–363, 2018

Keirsey D: The myth of mental illness. Professor Keirsey's Blog, July 26, 2011. Available at: https://professorkeirsey.wordpress.com/2011/07/26/the-myth-of-mental-illness. Accessed July 24, 2020.

Kelly BD, Bracken P, Cavendish H, et al: The Myth of Mental Illness: 50 years after publication: what does it mean today? Irish J Psychol Med 27(1):35–43, 2010

Kramer M: Long-range studies of mental hospital patients: an important area for research in chronic disease. Milbank Q 83(4), 2005

Livingston JD, Boyd JE: Correlates and consequences of internalized stigma for people living with mental illness: a systematic review and meta-analysis. Soc Sci Med 71(12):2150–2161, 2010

Mark TL, Levit KR, Buck JA: Datapoints: psychotropic drug prescriptions by medical specialty. Psychiatr Serv 60(9):1167, 2009

Maugh THII: Dr. Thomas Szasz dies at 92; psychiatrist who attacked profession. Los Angeles Times, September 17, 2012. Available at: www.latimes.com/local/obituaries/la-me-thomas-szasz-20120917-1-story.html. Accessed July 24, 2020.

McCance-Katz EF: The federal government ignores the treatment needs of Americans with serious mental illness. Psychiatric Times, Apr 21, 2016. Available at: www.psychiatrictimes.com/depression/federal-government-ignores-treatment-needs-americans-serious-mental-illness. Accessed July 24, 2020.

McGinty EE, Kennedy-Hendricks A, Choksy S, et al: Trends in news media coverage of mental illness in the United States: 1995–2014. Health Aff (Millwood) 35(6):1121–1129, 2016

McGorry PD, Purcell R, Goldstone S, et al: Age of onset and timing of treatment for mental and substance use disorders: implications for preventive intervention strategies and models of care. Curr Opin Psychiatry 24(4):301–306, 2011

Menninger RW: The therapeutic environment and team approach at the Menninger Hospital. Psychiatry Clin Neurosci 52(suppl):S173–S176, 1998

Phillips J, Frances A, Cerullo MA, et al: The six most essential questions in psychiatric diagnosis: a pluralogue part 1: conceptual and definitional issues in psychiatric diagnosis. Philos Ethics Humanit Med 7(1):3, 2012

Pilgrim D: The survival of psychiatric diagnosis. Soc Sci Med 65(3):536–547, 2007

Rissmiller DJ, Rissmiller JH: Open forum: evolution of the antipsychiatry movement into mental health consumerism. Psychiatr Serv 57(6):863–866, 2006

Sawada N, Uchida H, Suzuki T, et al: Persistence and compliance to antidepressant treatment in patients with depression: a chart review. BMC Psychiatry 9(1):38, 2009

Schwarz A: ADHD Nation: Children, Doctors, Big Pharma, and the Making of an American Epidemic. New York, Scribner, 2016

Shepherd GM: Creating Modern Neuroscience: The Revolutionary 1950s. New York, Oxford University Press, 2009

Substance Abuse and Mental Health Services Administration: Key Substance Use and Mental Health Indicators in the United States: Results From the 2017 National Survey on Drug Use and Health (HHS Publ No SMA-18-5068, NSDUH Series H-53). 2018. Available at: www.samhsa.gov/data/sites/default/files/cbhsq-reports/NSDUHFFR2017/NSDUHFFR2017.pdf. Accessed July 21, 2020.

Szalai J: Mental illness is all in your brain—or is it? New York Times, April 24, 2019. Available at: www.nytimes.com/2019/04/24/books/review-mind-fixers-psychiatry-biology-mental-illness-anne-harrington.html. Accessed July 24, 2020.

Szasz TS: The myth of mental illness. Am Psychol 15(2):113–118, 1960

Szasz TS: The Myth of Mental Illness: Foundations of a Theory of Personal Conduct. New York, Harper & Row, 1961

Szasz TS: Psychiatry: The Science of Lies. Syracuse, NY, Syracuse University Press, 2008

Torrey EF: Improving the mental health system: who is responsible? Psychiatric Times, December 24, 2014. Available at: www.psychiatrictimes.com/cultural-psychiatry/improving-mental-health-system-who-responsible. Accessed July 24, 2020.

Universal Health Services: Poll examining Americans' perceptions on mental health. March 12, 2019. Available at: www.multivu.com/players/English/8493951-uhs-americans-perceptions-of-mental-health-poll. Accessed July 24, 2020.

Urban Dictionary: Shrink. Gumba Gumba, April 6, 2004. Available at: www.urbandictionary.com/define.php?term=shrink. Accessed July 24, 2020.

Wang PS, Berglund P, Olfson M, et al: Failure and delay in initial treatment contact after first onset of mental disorders in the National Comorbidity Survey Replication. Arch Gen Psychiatry 62(6):603–613, 2005

Whitaker R: Anatomy of an Epidemic: Magic Bullets, Psychiatric Drugs, and the Astonishing Rise of Mental Illness in America. New York, Broadway Books, 2010

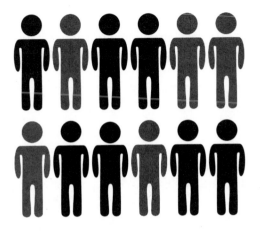

Mental Illness Is Real

Half Truth: We do not know exactly what causes mental illnesses.

Whole Truth: Although we do not know exactly what causes mental illnesses, we do know that mental illness is biological illness.

Important Points

- We can show biological abnormalities with all the major mental illnesses.
- We can show brain abnormalities with head scans, microscopic studies, and neurotransmitter studies.
- We can show abnormalities in the rest of the body with genetic studies, hormone studies, inflammation studies, and studies of the gut.

- Although we do not know a vast amount about what causes mental illness, we know more than enough to be sure it is physical illness.

Introduction

If the human brain is the most complex of all organs, then the pathology of mental illnesses is destined to be the most complex field in all of medicine. Because of this complexity, and because we lack a central pathophysiology for each of the major mental illnesses, no clinician can feel fully confident in speaking of the biology of mental illness. No clinician can keep pace with the vast and rapidly developing field of neuropathology, much less with neuroscience generally. Only a subspecialist in one major disorder (such as obsessive-compulsive disorder or schizophrenia) can remain conversant in all the research and the most current neurobiological theories.

Nevertheless, all clinicians can feel confident that the major mental illnesses are biologically and medically real, and all of us need to be prepared to say so both inside and outside of the consulting room. We need to remember that we do not need to explain the central pathophysiology of mental illness or the intricacies of the latest research. Instead, we need to show that mental illness is biologically based. For this, we only need a few examples from the wealth of research showing neurological and other physical changes with mental illness. By showing atrophy due to mental illness on head scans, or loss of brain cells with microscopic studies, or increased levels of inflammation early in mental illnesses, we can demonstrate that mental illness is medically real. For advocates, simpler and more intuitive examples are vastly more effective than sophisticated discourses for expressing what we want to convey: Mental illnesses are biologically and medically real.

Mental Illness Is Medical

Dr. Thomas Szasz (1961) claimed that if mental illness is not biological, it is not real (see Chapter 4). His challenge remains at the core of criticisms about psychiatry and mental illness, and it should. Critics should demand that only medical illnesses should be treated as medically. Mental illness that is not also physical is a contradiction in terms, and misleading. Worse than that, false diagnosis of mental illness only confuses people who are struggling with life, and leads them into dead ends when they seek solutions. It leads them to powerful and expensive medical treatments that would make them worse rather than better. If mental illness is not medical, then psychiatry really is the monstrous crime that some critics claim. That would mean that thousands of people are hospitalized right now for no good reason, law courts are taking away their freedoms for no good reason, millions of people are taking powerful medicines for no good reason, and everyone is paying higher taxes and insurance premiums for no good reason. Mental health care costs $108 billion a year in this country (Bureau of Economic Analysis, U.S. Department of Commerce 2019). If there is no such thing as medical mental illness, then all of this represents a fraud of unprecedented historic proportions.

This book is in your hands because today we can answer Dr. Szasz's challenge. In the 1960s, no one could refute Dr. Szasz. But today, we can answer his questions in just the way he demanded: We can show that mental illness is true biological dysfunction. Mental illness is medical as well as mental, and we can prove it. We can scan the brain of someone with schizophrenia or depression or any other major mental illness and show that the brain is not functioning normally. We can put a brain under a microscope and see nerve cells shriveling and dying. We can show widespread changes in normal neurotransmitter activity throughout the brain. We can show how genes physically put people at risk for mental illness, and how stress can trigger that risk. We can show that hormones, inflammation, and immune function are affected all over the brain and body during mental illness.

The science behind these claims is now overwhelming. We do not have only a few or even a few hundred studies that show the biological reality of mental illness. We have thousands and thousands of legitimate, solid scientific studies that show this reality in a variety of ways. We have so many studies that no one person could read them all. Everything that I present in the rest of this book is well established by scores of studies. Nothing I discuss is brand-new or especially controversial. It is just straightforward biological and medical science, using the same standards of legitimacy that are used in other branches of medicine. Yes, mental illness also involves a mental level of reality that is not always present with other kinds of illnesses. Mental events can cause mental illness, and mental treatments can treat mental illness. But in the next two chapters we will focus on the physical level of mental illness. And investigating the physical level of mental illness uses the same science as the rest of medicine and biology. See for yourself.

Head Scan Studies: Worth a Thousand Words

When *The Myth of Mental Illness* was published, no one could look inside the brain of a living person. Doctors could see broken bones with X-rays, heart attacks with electrocardiograms (ECGs), and ear infections with otoscopes. But there was no way to look into a living brain to physically diagnose whether mental illness was present.

In the late 1970s, the situation began to change. Computed tomography (CT) scans made it possible to take pictures of living brain tissue. Magnetic resonance imaging (MRI) followed, with even better images. Then "functional imaging" allowed us to see the activity of the living brain. This emerged in the 1980s with single-photon emission computed tomography (SPECT) and positron emission tomography (PET) scans, followed in the 1990s by functional MRI (fMRI). Differences between these methods are not as important as the fact that researchers could now see levels of high and low activity in the brain, and track the use of oxygen, glucose (blood sugar), and other important chemicals (Raichle 2009). All of these showed us extraordinary things about the brain, and neuroscience has never looked back.

Structural Imaging

What have we learned about mental illnesses? Out of the thousands of studies published, let's look at a few examples. First, CT and MRI scans can show structural changes in the brain—changes in the physical size and shape of various parts of the brain. If we can see that brain tissue shrinks (atrophies) or is lost during mental illness, then we have evidence that mental illness physically affects the brain.

Does mental illness change the size and shape of the brain? Yes. How do we know? Consider one scientific review that analyzed 193 well-done studies involving 15,892 people, comparing brains of those with mental illness to those with no mental illness. Results showed clear losses of gray matter, the brain tissue that contains the bodies of nerve cells. (Gray matter is found on the outside surface—the cortex—of the brain, and white matter on much of the inside. White matter is composed of the connections between nerve cells.) The gray matter losses specifically occurred in parts of the brain that regulate our emotions and thinking. Furthermore, the most severe form of mental illness (psychosis) was accompanied by the greatest losses of brain tissue. In the case of schizophrenia, studies showed that brain tissue losses occur as the illness develops. These changes in brain tissue are not due to psychiatric medications. They are due to mental illness (Goodkind et al. 2015).

Functional Imaging

Imaging can be used to see mental illness as it changes the *shape* of the brain, but it is just as important to show how mental illness changes the *functioning* of the brain. We can see this change on PET, SPECT, and fMRI scans. The results are extremely complex, as we would expect. The brain is the most

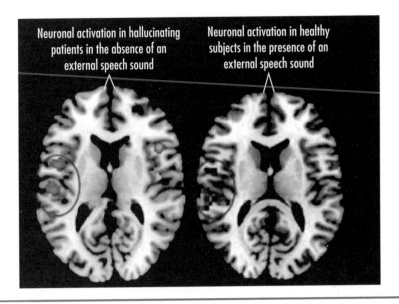

FIGURE 5–1. Brain activations in individuals hallucinating compared with those hearing actual voices.

To view this figure in color, see Plate 1 in Color Gallery.

On the right, you can see a normal brain. The circled area activates in the presence of actual voices. On the left, you can see the brain of someone hallucinating a voice. The same circled area activates in the absence of an exterior voice.

Source. Reprinted from Hugdahl K: "Auditory Hallucinations: A Review of the ERC 'VOICE' Project." *World Journal of Psychiatry* 5(2):193–209, 2015. Used with permission.

complex object in the physical universe, and head scans confirm this. Although thousands of studies have been done, thousands more will be required to show the precise nature of each mental illness. However, we have more than enough evidence right now to show that mental illness is real. One example is schizophrenia. Researchers looked at people having auditory hallucinations—for instance, hearing voices when no one is around. They found that when people hear hallucinated voices, the same part of the brain lights up as when people hear real voices. Why do people with schizophrenia hear voices? Because the brain region for processing voices activates when there are no voices around. This may seem obvious, but that is only if we already understand mental illness as physical illness. The brain is not behaving normally, and you can see it for yourself on head scans (Hugdahl 2015) (Figure 5–1).

Here is another example: People with addiction suffer from a devastating, often fatal illness. Can we show that their brains are functioning abnormally?

Yes, and in many different ways. One of these is found in the brain's reward center, called the *nucleus accumbens*. The reward center is located deep in the brain, as you can see in Figure 5–2. The nucleus accumbens activates when we think of something we want. It gives us a feeling of positive motivation and craving for things we desire, whether they are food, drink, sex, video games, or even knowledge. This feeling of desire and motivation corresponds to dopamine release in the nucleus accumbens. When we come across something desirable, it is dopamine that activates the reward center, telling us that this is something we want. Dopamine is important for normal human motivation. But drugs of abuse cause *abnormal* amounts of dopamine release in the nucleus accumbens. This causes overwhelming levels of desire for substances above all other rewards. These unnatural levels of dopamine release also cause the reward center to respond less and less to normal rewards. As a result, people with addiction gradually lose interest in all other parts of life. Their brains have been hijacked by the drug, and do not care about anything but getting more of it. This is the same idea as in the famous experiments in which rats relentlessly pressed a lever for cocaine, ignoring food and every other reward until they literally died of cocaine use (Wise and Koob 2014). When we look at brain scans of humans, it turns out that people with addiction have abnormally low levels of dopamine responsiveness in the reward center, corresponding to their lack of motivation for normal rewards (Volkow et al. 2007, 2009). You can see this in Figure 5–2.

These are only two examples out of hundreds from studies of all the major mental illnesses, such as major depression, bipolar disorder (manic-depression), and obsessive-compulsive disorder (OCD). But the science of mental illness is vast and goes well beyond head scans, so let's look at some other kinds of studies.

Genetic Studies: A Family Affair

Most people realize that mental illness runs in families. We can trace addiction and depression, for example, through many generations of some families. But this knowledge alone does not tell us whether mental illness is also physical. Clearly, people can learn ways of feeling, thinking, and behaving, and children growing up in families are exquisitely sensitive to this kind of learning. So how do we know whether the mental illness is physical, from genes, or mental, from learning?

In general, we know that mental illness results from both genes and learning. It is not one or the other, but both. The question here is whether we can

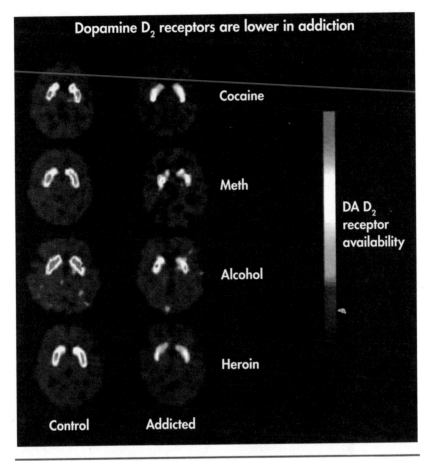

FIGURE 5–2. Dopamine receptors in the nucleus accumbens, the brain's reward center.

To view this figure in color, see Plate 2 in Color Gallery.

On the left are normal (control) brains, while on the right are brains of people with addiction. There are fewer dopamine (DA) receptors and there is less response to dopamine in people with addicted brains, as shown by brighter, larger areas of activity in the "normal" brains on the left.

Source. National Institute on Drug Abuse: "NIDA's Newest Division Mines Clinical Applications From Basic Research." October 1, 2007. Available at: https://archives.drugabuse.gov/news-events/nida-notes/2007/10/nidas-newest-division-mines-clinical-applications-basic-research. Accessed July 27, 2020.

show that there is a strong physical inheritance through the genes contained in someone's DNA. There are two obvious ways of doing this, and they both involve twins: One way is to study twins adopted into different families and compare them with twins growing up in the same family. Another way is to compare identical (monozygotic) twins with fraternal (dizygotic) twins. Identical twins have 100% of their DNA in common, whereas fraternal twins have 50% of their DNA in common, as do all brothers and sisters who are not identical twins. So any familial illness that is passed on should show up more in both identical twins than in both fraternal twins. This would show that the illness is physical and transmitted (in part) by genes.

What do we find? Genetic studies indeed show that mental illness is transmitted physically through genes. In Figure 5–3, you can see that the more DNA two people share, the more likely they are to share the illness of schizophrenia. If one identical twin has schizophrenia, there is about a 50% chance that the other will as well. On the other hand, if one fraternal twin has schizophrenia, there is about a 17% chance that the other will, about the same risk as for any other pair of brothers or sisters. The closer the family relationship, the higher the risk of schizophrenia. When we get to very distant relationships, like second cousins, the risk is so low that it approaches 1%, the same risk as in the general population (Riley and Kendler 2006).

We find similar results regarding alcoholism, a common form of addiction. Twin and adoption studies show that there is a moderate to high contribution of genetics to the risk for alcoholism, in addition to any family environment and cultural influences (Agrawal and Lynskey 2008; Kendler et al. 1992). We can also show strong genetic contributions to bipolar disorder, major depression, anxiety disorders, and many more. Studies even show that attention-deficit/hyperactivity disorder (ADHD) is 70%–80% due to genetics, which is a higher rate than for most other mental and physical conditions (Brikell et al. 2015). In fact, genes are a bigger contributing factor in ADHD than in diseases such as breast cancer (Möller et al. 2016), high blood pressure (Waken et al. 2017), or heart disease (McPherson and Tybjaerg-Hansen 2016). As is true of other mental health conditions, the risk is physically present in our genes, but it has to be activated by experience. And it turns out that experiences like stress are capable of physically turning on and off genes related to mental illness. Experiences, even mental events, modify the brain, all the way down to which genes get activated and when they are activated. So it is really not surprising that genes and their expression are a big part of mental illness (Kandel 1998). In this sense, mental abnormalities and physical abnormalities always go together.

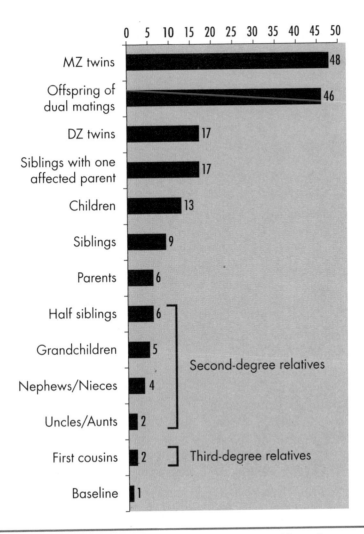

FIGURE 5–3. Rates of schizophrenia (percentages) based on genetic relationships.

The highest rates of schizophrenia (nearly 50%) are found among those who share all of their genes with others who have schizophrenia, like children of parents who both have the disorder (listed in figure as "offspring of dual matings") or identical twins. As a relative with schizophrenia becomes more distant, the risk of the disease goes does. So having a first cousin with schizophrenia only carries a risk of 2%.

DZ=dizygotic; MZ=monozygotic.

Source. Reprinted from Riley B, Kendler KS: "Molecular Genetic Studies of Schizophrenia." *European Journal of Human Genetics* 14(6):669–680, 2006. Used with permission.

Cellular Disease: Mental Illness Under the Microscope

Another way of looking at medical illness is through microscopic studies. This is a time-honored part of medicine. In fact, my father was a doctor who trained in the early 1960s. He remembers being on call in the middle of the night and running samples of urine and sputum directly to the microscope, where he would look for signs of bacterial infections and other common conditions. Though things are infinitely more complicated with mental illness, we can still examine mental illness on a microscopic level. And here, too, we find evidence of physical illness.

One example involves major depression. Some people believe that major depression is just a form of normal sadness and grief, that we should not call it a disease. However, the microscopic level tells its own story. In major depression, microscopic studies show many areas of the brain affected. One area of change involves the hippocampus, located deep within each temporal lobe.

The hippocampus is vital to memory and emotion regulation, and the hippocampus shrinks to a smaller size in major depression (as well as in other illnesses, such as posttraumatic stress disorder [PTSD] [Figure 5–4]). Microscopic evidence shows that in depression, nerve cells die faster and develop more slowly than normal. There is a marked downturn in neurogenesis (the production of new neurons). There is also a lack of sprouting and growing in neurons. You can imagine these differences as being similar to plants: Unhealthy plants shrivel and die, whereas healthy ones sprout and grow. Neurons act the same way. In fact, the brain has its own equivalents of plant food, and one important one is a growth-causing chemical called brain-derived neurotrophic factor (BDNF). In depression, expression or levels of BDNF are abnormally low, corresponding to a lack of new growth among nerve cells. This is profoundly important, but what is even more important is that the hippocampus can regrow through treatment with antidepressant medications. There is scientific evidence that antidepressants actually increase BDNF and its effects, promoting healing in the brain (Lee and Kim 2010; Liu et al. 2017). Healing that we can see.

Neurotransmitters and Other Troublesome Chemicals

BDNF is not the only chemical that becomes unbalanced during depression. Abnormalities of serotonin, dopamine, and norepinephrine also occur. Al-

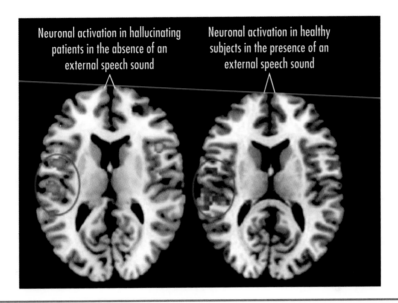

PLATE 1. *(Figure 5–1)* Brain activations in individuals hallucinating compared with those hearing actual voices.

On the right, you can see a normal brain. The circled area activates in the presence of actual voices. On the left, you can see the brain of someone hallucinating a voice. The same circled area activates in the absence of an exterior voice.

Source. Reprinted from Hugdahl K: "Auditory Hallucinations: A Review of the ERC 'VOICE' Project." *World Journal of Psychiatry* 5(2):193–209, 2015. Used with permission.

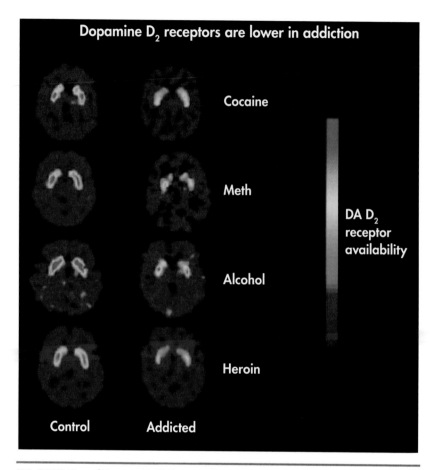

PLATE 2. *(Figure 5–2)* Dopamine receptors in the nucleus accumbens, the brain's reward center.

On the left are normal (control) brains, while on the right are brains of people with addiction. There are fewer dopamine (DA) receptors and there is less response to dopamine in people with addicted brains, as shown by brighter, larger areas of activity in the "normal" brains on the left.

Source. National Institute on Drug Abuse: "NIDA's Newest Division Mines Clinical Applications From Basic Research." October 1, 2007. Available at: https://archives.drugabuse.gov/news-events/nida-notes/2007/10/nidas-newest-division-mines-clinical-applications-basic-research. Accessed July 27, 2020.

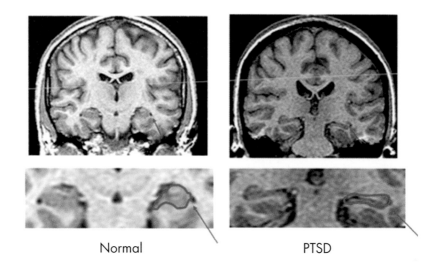

Normal　　　　　　　　　PTSD

PLATE 3. *(Figure 5–4)* An example of shrinking brain tissue (atrophy) due to PTSD.

The shaded area in each picture is the hippocampus. The hippocampus is smaller than normal in PTSD.

Source. Campbell and MacQueen 2004; Kitayama et al. 2005. Picture courtesy of Dr. Doug Bremner, Emory University.

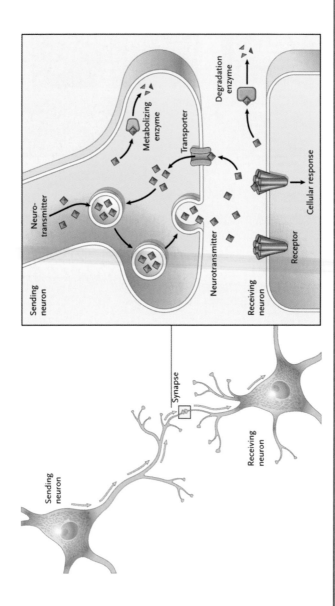

PLATE 4. *(Figure 5–5)* Neurotransmitters: chemical molecules that carry messages from one neuron to the next.

The picture on the left shows two neurons with a close connection (synapse). On the right, the picture zooms in to the end of one neuron and the beginning of another. It shows neurotransmitters being released by the neuron above and binding to the receiving neuron below.

Source. National Institute on Drug Abuse (National Institutes of Health).

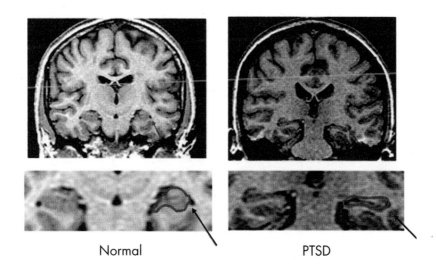

Normal   PTSD

FIGURE 5–4. An MRI scan of shrinking brain tissue (atrophy) due to PTSD.

To view this figure in color, see Plate 3 in Color Gallery.

The shaded area in each picture is the hippocampus. The hippocampus is often smaller than normal in PTSD. This can occur in major depression as well.

Source. Campbell and MacQueen 2004; Kitayama et al. 2005. Picture courtesy of Dr. Doug Bremner, Emory University.

though these chemicals do not tell us the whole story about depression and other mental illnesses, there is good evidence that they do play a role (Belmaker and Agam 2008). All three are important neurotransmitters, the chemical messengers that carry signals from one neuron to another (Figure 5–5).

Researchers have illustrated neurotransmitter changes in a number of interesting experiments on depression. In one type of study, people took pills to artificially deplete either serotonin or norepinephrine. This had little effect in "normals" (healthy control subjects), but people who had used antidepressants to recover from depression relapsed back into depression (Ruhé et al. 2007).

Similar sorts of experiments have been done to study abnormalities in patients with panic disorder. For instance, there is good evidence that people with panic attacks are abnormally sensitive to norepinephrine, the body's chemical messenger of fear. Small amounts of this chemical trigger panic attacks in people with panic disorder, but not in people without it. Interestingly, people with panic attacks are abnormally sensitive to a number of other substances as well. Inhaling air with extra carbon dioxide (CO_2)

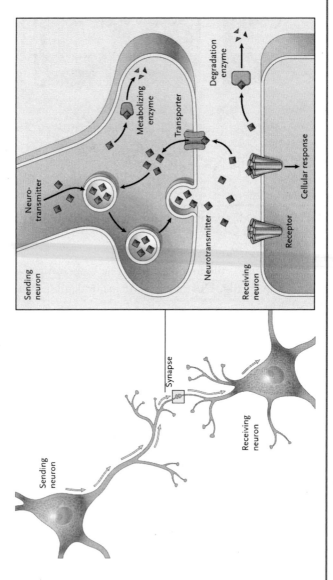

FIGURE 5–5. Neurotransmitters: chemical molecules that carry messages from one neuron to the next.
*To view this figure in color, see **Plate 4 in Color Gallery.***
The picture on the left shows two neurons with a close connection (synapse). On the right, the picture zooms in to the end of one neuron and the beginning of another. It shows neurotransmitters being released by the neuron above and binding to the receiving neuron below.
Source.   National Institute on Drug Abuse (National Institutes of Health).

triggers panic attacks in people with panic disorder, but not in those without the disorder. This occurs even if the people with panic attacks do not know whether they are breathing in extra CO_2. Why should the rest of us care? Because these kinds of experiments illustrate the physical nature of mental illness. Even when people with the illness do not mentally know that it is happening, chemical signals in the body can trigger a relapse of the symptoms. If panic disorder and major depression were only mental, then these results would be impossible. Hundreds of experiments support these findings (Bandelow et al. 2017; Johnson et al. 2014), and hundreds of other experiments have documented neurotransmitter changes in other mental disorders, including every major mental illness.

Mental Illness and the Rest of the Body

All of this barely scratches the surface of research on psychiatric disorders, but it repeatedly shows that mental illness is also biological illness. Mental illness is certainly brain illness, but it is more than brain illness. Mental illness is also illness of the whole body. We will look at what mental health disorders do to the body in the next chapter, and find devastating results. In this one, we discuss how mental illness changes the body, including hormones, inflammation, and even digestion.

Hormones

Hormones are chemical messengers that go all over the body to regulate bodily functions. For instance, thyroid hormone regulates the rate of metabolism, whereas sex hormones such as testosterone and estrogen regulate sexual function. Are hormones affected in mental illness? In many cases, they are. For instance, thyroid abnormalities are more common in individuals who have bipolar disorder (Chakrabarti 2011). And women with schizophrenia seem to have lower estrogen levels; this would fit with the fact that estrogen seems to be protective against schizophrenia, and helps explain why schizophrenia is more common in men than women (Gogos et al. 2015). Estrogen has many other effects on the brain (McEwen et al. 2012). For instance, women become more vulnerable to major depression when they go through puberty, when they have children, and when they go through menopause—these are the times when estrogen changes the most and the times when women get depressed the most.

One hormone that is intimately related to many mental illnesses is cortisol (Zorn et al. 2017). This makes sense because cortisol is one of our main stress hormones, and illnesses such as depression and PTSD involve abnormally high levels of stress. Cortisol and the stress hormone system are altered in these disorders, and in a variety of ways. For instance, cortisol levels run higher in major depression and lower in PTSD (Lopez-Duran et al. 2009; Morris et al. 2012; Stetler and Miller 2011). People with depression tend to be negative and stressed most of the time, and this correlates with higher levels of cortisol. In PTSD, the brain appears abnormally sensitive to cortisol and acts as if it is trying to suppress cortisol release. In both cases, the body's hormone system is not functioning correctly. And in both cases, the picture is complex, with many differences between individuals. Nevertheless, there are hundreds of studies documenting stress hormone dysfunction in these disorders. And while brain abnormalities cause hormone dysfunction, cortisol dysfunction in turn has negative effects on the brain. Cortisol also raises blood sugar, lowers immunity, and causes weight gain, among other things. A vicious cycle develops between brain dysfunction and hormone dysfunction in these disorders, taking a toll on both body and brain.

Inflammation

Inflammation is one of the most exciting areas of current medical research. Scientists have found that inflammation plays an important role in causing common illnesses such as diabetes and heart disease. Inflammation also has a role in mental illness. What is inflammation? Inflammation is the body's response to a threat. This threat usually takes the form of infection or injury. In either case, inflammation is the body's way of activating to fight off infection and promote healing. White blood cells are activated, and chemicals such as interleukin 6 (IL-6), C-reactive protein (CRP), and tumor necrosis factor (TNF) are released throughout the body. These chemicals act as signals for the body to go into self-defense mode. Meanwhile, inflammation makes people slow down and take time to heal. Inflammation causes people to feel tired and achy when they are sick, often making them want to stay in bed and do nothing.

Interestingly, the body releases many of the same inflammatory chemicals in mental illness. In major depression, for example, people also feel tired and achy, lacking motivation to do much of anything, including physical or social activity. They feel like they are sick, and in fact they are. Studies have shown that inflammatory and immune responses overlap in major depression and other illnesses such as a cold or the flu. Chemicals such as

IL-6, CRP, and TNF are increased in depression, as in other common illnesses, resulting in lower levels of serotonin, dopamine, norepinephrine, and BDNF, which are also involved in depression. Although inflammation is not the sole cause of depression, it is one part of the picture, and is probably a big factor for some people and a small one for others (Miller and Raison 2016). Inflammation, however, has been proven to cause depressive symptoms. For instance, people who are given a chemical to trigger an immune response show a temporary dip in mood as their bodies mount a reaction. Even more interestingly, the most common time for people to die by suicide is not when the weather is darkest (during the winter, around the holidays) but in the spring. This pattern occurs all over the world, and spring happens to be when allergens are the highest worldwide. Researchers have argued that allergens increase inflammation, lowering mood and making desperate people even more desperate in these times (Amritwar et al. 2017).

Inflammation is also increased in individuals with bipolar disorder (Muneer 2016). One review identified 22 separate inflammatory factors, including CRP and IL-6, that are increased in bipolar disorder. There is evidence of inflammation both in the brain and in the rest of the body for people with this disorder (Fries et al. 2018). There is also strong evidence that inflammation is an important factor in schizophrenia, and researchers are actively investigating anti-inflammatory medications as treatment options (Khandaker et al. 2015; Müller 2018).

The Brain-Gut Connection

One cause of all that inflammation is known as "leaky gut syndrome." This sounds made-up, but it is scientifically real. Our digestive tract is full of bacteria, and stress (among many other factors) allows bacteria to leak into the rest of the body. This causes an immune reaction, which can increase inflammation all over the body. This, in turn, seems to increase our risk of mental illness (Miller and Raison 2016).

However, the gut-brain connection involves more than inflammation. Many of the same chemicals that transmit messages in the brain transmit them in the gut as well. For instance, most of the body's supply of serotonin is found along the gut, not in the brain. This is probably one reason that many people get an upset stomach or diarrhea when they are stressed. Also, the bacteria in our digestive tracts apparently have effects on our brains (Del Colle et al. 2020; Grenham et al. 2011).

Each of us carries around about 2 pounds of bacteria and other microorganisms. In fact, we have about 10 times more bacterial cells than human cells, and we need them to survive and function normally. Bacteria are necessary for digestion and immunity, but the brain also needs them (Rogers et al. 2016). They are capable of making serotonin, dopamine, BDNF, and many more substances that affect the brain. Some of them are helpful and some are hurtful, depending on the situation. In part, the helpful or hurtful effects depend on the particular mix of bacteria in our digestive systems. This information has led researchers to wonder whether probiotics—which provide people with particular species of bacteria to live in the gut—can help mental illnesses such as autism and bipolar disorder. A number of studies have already shown that probiotics may decrease anxiety and stress, lowering stress hormones in the process. And there is good evidence that people with autism, schizophrenia, depression, and bipolar disorder have altered mixes of bacteria in their digestive systems. So researchers are also studying whether probiotics can help ease symptoms of these disorders. The results are not yet ready for widespread use, but they are more than enough to justify further study (Genedi et al. 2019; Sarkar et al. 2016; Sharon et al. 2016; Zhou and Foster 2015).

Obviously, if gut bacteria do interact with mental illness, then mental illness must have a strong physical component. Bacteria cause other physical illnesses, such as pneumonia and bladder infections, and it appears that bacteria play some role in many mental illnesses. This would be impossible if mental illness were only mental and cultural. Yet changes in bacteria often result in changes in the body and brain, which can in turn develop into changes in the mind from mental illness. As human beings, we cannot separate mind from body, and we simply cannot separate mental illness from physical illness.

The Biology of Mental Illness: All Figured Out?

The evidence for the biology of mental illness is overwhelming. For every major mental illness, we have head scan studies, microscopic studies, neurotransmitter studies, genetic studies, hormone studies, and inflammation studies. We have hundreds, sometimes thousands, of these studies in each category. You can see it for yourself, both in this book and any time you care to do an internet search. You can see pictures and charts of brain tissue loss, brain dysfunction, hormone changes, and inflammation that go along with mental illness. There is simply no current ongoing scientific debate as to whether mental illness is a form of physical illness. Medical researchers in all branches of medicine accept that mental illness is physical. The debate was settled long ago, and research has moved on to understanding how the brain is malfunctioning in mental illness, and how mental illness interacts with the rest of the body.

At the same time, with all this amazing knowledge, people wonder why we don't have mental illness all figured out. Why don't we just do a head scan to diagnose schizophrenia or PTSD? Why not do a lab test to measure inflammation or hormones, so that we can diagnose and treat these illnesses with medical precision? Why don't we have medical cures for all these illnesses, if we know so much about their biology?

In truth, we *know* a vast amount about the biology of mental illness, and we also *don't know* a vast amount about the biology of mental illness. The brain is the most complicated thing there is, and it is exquisitely difficult to figure out just what goes wrong in any mental illness. In some cases, such as Alzheimer's dementia, we can make a diagnosis using head scans. But those head scans are not so much better than talking to a psychiatrist that it is worth thousands of dollars to do them. This is an important point: Psychiatrists and other trained professionals are actually good at diagnosing mental illness using their brains. Put another way, the human brain is still the best tool professionals have for diagnosing illnesses of the human brain, so lab tests need to be significantly better to justify the cost. Also, although we can test for hormone and inflammatory levels, we should only do so when it will change the treatment. In most cases, the treatment is the same regardless of the lab results. At the same time, lab testing with mental illness is becoming more common all the time. For instance, we now have useful DNA tests to help us select a medication and match the medication to the biology of each individual patient. Certainly, lab tests and head scans are going to be common diagnostic tools in the future. Right now, they are standard research tools but only occasional diagnostic tools (Rosenblat et al. 2017). They can easily tell us about the biological realities of mental illness, but overall, they are not better than human beings at diagnosing it.

Although biological *diagnosis* is still under development, biological *research* is well developed. We don't know enough to specify every microscopic step in the development of a mental illness, but we know more than enough to be sure mental illness is real medical illness. Today, there is so much biological research on mental illness and the brain that no one person could read it all in a lifetime. Thousands of new studies are published every year. It would take many volumes to discuss all of the new research and treatment possibilities for even one of the major mental illnesses. I have discussed a few examples here, but I have not even mentioned most mental illnesses and the science behind them. For instance, we have extensive knowledge of the biology of Alzheimer's dementia, obsessive-compulsive disorder, anorexia nervosa, borderline personality disorder, and many more.

Although we know with certainty that mental illness is biological, we do not know precisely how each mental illness works or how it can be cured. Why is this? The problem is not finding evidence that mental illness is biological. The problem is putting together the overwhelming amount of biological data into a complete picture for each illness. It is not going to be simple. As of today, we cannot put all the data, all the pieces of the puzzle, into one neat picture. Given that this puzzle (the brain) has about 100 billion pieces, that is to be expected. On the other hand, there is a simpler way to show that mental illness is physical. In the next chapter we will look at the ways that mental illness has all the devastating consequences of any other kind of medical illness. And we will see what everyone who has ever experienced it already knows: Mental illness is terrifyingly real.

Advice for Advocacy

- Pictures are useful to powerfully convey this material. Pictures allow people to see for themselves and make up their own minds. This is entirely different from hearing a recognized expert assert the same thing.
- Biological and medical realities are the things we can see, touch, and point toward. Pictures of head scans, cartoons of neurons and neurotransmitters, and graphs of genetic relationships will unarguably convey the physical realities of mental functioning and mental illness.
- The simplest examples are the best. I have attempted to provide some in this chapter.
- You do not need to explain the pathophysiology of even one mental illness. You do not need to put yourself forward as an expert in neuroscience. Instead, you simply need to open a window into the fascinating world of brain science and gaze in wonder, along with everyone else, as you present just a bit of what goes on in people's brains when they are depressed, or anxious, or psychotic.
- Depending on the time available, one to three examples can be followed by a general assertion that we have hundreds, even thousands, of head scan studies, microscopic studies, genetic studies, and neurotransmitter studies on mental illness. Doubters can easily confirm this using internet search engines.
- If people have residual doubts about the biology of mental illness, presenting whole body effects can be profoundly persuasive. Thus, it is helpful to show an example or two of the ways

that mental illnesses can increase levels of inflammation, influence hormone function, or increase risks of diabetes and heart disease.

- It may not be possible to convince everyone with this material alone. These studies bring up a host of complex and sometimes irresolvable questions. But rhetorically, this material can open the undeniable possibility that mental illness is real, while the material presented in Chapter 6 can clinch the argument: Mental illness is medically real because it is deadly, disabling, and physically devastating.

References

Agrawal A, Lynskey MT: Are there genetic influences on addiction: evidence from family, adoption and twin studies. Addiction 103(7):1069–1081, 2008

Amritwar AU, Lowry CA, Brenner LA, et al: Mental health in allergic rhinitis: depression and suicidal behavior. Curr Treat Options Allergy 4(1):71–97, 2017

Bandelow B, Baldwin D, Abelli M, et al: Biological markers for anxiety disorders, OCD and PTSD: a consensus statement. Part II: neurochemistry, neurophysiology and neurocognition. World J Biol Psychiatry 18(3):162–214, 2017

Belmaker RH, Agam G: Major depressive disorder. N Engl J Med 358(1):55–68, 2008

Brikell I, Kuja-Halkola R, Larsson H: Heritability of attention-deficit hyperactivity disorder in adults. Am J Med Genet B Neuropsychiatr Genet 168(6):406–413, 2015

Bureau of Economic Analysis, U.S. Department of Commerce: 2015 Blended Account Release Table. March 5, 2019. Available at: www.bea.gov/system/files/2019-03/2015-Blended-Account-Release-Table.xlsx. Retrieved September 12, 2019.

Campbell S, MacQueen G: The role of the hippocampus in the pathophysiology of major depression. J Psychiatry Neurosci 29(6):417–426, 2004

Chakrabarti S: Thyroid functions and bipolar affective disorder. J Thyroid Res 2011:306367, 2011

Del Colle A, Israelyan N, Gross Margolis K: Novel aspects of enteric serotonergic signaling in health and brain-gut disease. Am J Physiology Gastrointest Liver Physiol 318(1):G130–143, 2020

Fries GR, Walss-Bass C, Bauer ME, et al: Revisiting inflammation in bipolar disorder. Pharmacol Biochem Behav 177:12–19, 2018

Genedi M, Janmaat IE, Haarman BB, et al: Dysregulation of the gut-brain axis in schizophrenia and bipolar disorder: probiotic supplementation as a supportive treatment in psychiatric disorders. Curr Opin Psychiatry 32(3):185–195, 2019

Gogos A, Sbisa AM, Sun J, et al: A role for estrogen in schizophrenia: clinical and preclinical findings. Int J Endocrinol 2015:615356, 2015

Goodkind M, Eickhoff SB, Oathes DJ, et al: Identification of a common neurobiological substrate for mental illness. JAMA Psychiatry 72(4):305–315, 2015

Grenham S, Clarke G, Cryan JF, Dinan TG: Brain-gut–microbe communication in health and disease. Front Physiol 2:94, 2011

Hugdahl K: Auditory hallucinations: a review of the ERC "VOICE" project. World J Psychiatry 5(2):193–209, 2015

Johnson PL, Federici LM, Shekhar A: Etiology, triggers and neurochemical circuits associated with unexpected, expected, and laboratory-induced panic attacks. Neurosci Biobehav Rev 46 (Pt 3):429–454, 2014

Kandel ER: A new intellectual framework for psychiatry. Am J Psychiatry155(4):457–469, 1998

Kendler KS, Heath AC, Neale MC, et al: A population-based twin study of alcoholism in women. JAMA 268(14):1877–1882, 1992

Khandaker GM, Cousins L, Deakin J, et al: Inflammation and immunity in schizophrenia: implications for pathophysiology and treatment. Lancet Psychiatry 2(3):258–270, 2015

Kitayama N, Vaccarino V, Kutner M, et al: Magnetic resonance imaging (MRI) measurement of hippocampal volume in posttraumatic stress disorder: a meta-analysis. J Affect Disord 88(1):79–86, 2005

Lee BH, Kim YK: The roles of BDNF in the pathophysiology of major depression and in antidepressant treatment. Psychiatry Invest 7(4):231–235, 2010

Liu W, Ge T, Leng Y, et al: The role of neural plasticity in depression: from hippocampus to prefrontal cortex. Neural Plast 2017:6871089, 2017

Lopez-Duran NL, Kovacs M, George CJ: Hypothalamic-pituitary-adrenal axis dysregulation in depressed children and adolescents: a meta-analysis. Psychoneuroendocrinology 34(9):1272–1283, 2009

McEwen BS, Akama KT, Spencer-Segal JL, et al: Estrogen effects on the brain: actions beyond the hypothalamus via novel mechanisms. Behav Neurosci 126(1):4–16, 2012

McPherson R, Tybjaerg-Hansen A: Genetics of coronary artery disease. Circ Res 118(4):564–578, 2016

Miller AH, Raison CL: The role of inflammation in depression: from evolutionary imperative to modern treatment target. Nat Rev Immunol 16(1):22–34, 2016

Möller S, Mucci LA, Harris JR, et al: The heritability of breast cancer among women in the Nordic Twin Study of Cancer. Cancer Biomarkers Prev 25(1):145–150, 2016

Morris MC, Compas BE, Garber J: Relations among posttraumatic stress disorder, comorbid major depression, and HPA function: a systematic review and meta-analysis. Clin Psychol Rev 32(4):301–315, 2012

Müller N: Inflammation in schizophrenia: pathogenetic aspects and therapeutic considerations. Schizophr Bull 44(5):973–982, 2018

Muneer A: Bipolar disorder: role of inflammation and the development of disease biomarkers. Psychiatry Investig 13(1):18–33, 2016

Raichle ME: A brief history of human brain mapping. Trends Neurosci 32(2):118–126, 2009

Riley B, Kendler KS: Molecular genetic studies of schizophrenia. Eur J Hum Genet 14(6):669–680, 2006

Rogers GB, Keating DJ, Young RL, et al: From gut dysbiosis to altered brain function and mental illness: mechanisms and pathways. Mol Psychiatry 21(6):738–748, 2016

Rosenblat JD, Lee Y, McIntyre RS: Does pharmacogenomic testing improve clinical outcomes for major depressive disorder? A systematic review of clinical trials and cost-effectiveness studies. J Clin Psychiatry 78(6):720–729, 2017

Ruhé HG, Mason NS, Schene AH: Mood is indirectly related to serotonin, norepinephrine and dopamine levels in humans: a meta-analysis of monoamine depletion studies. Mol Psychiatry 12(4):331–359, 2007

Sarkar A, Lehto SM, Harty S, et al: Psychobiotics and the manipulation of bacteria-gut-brain signals. Trends Neurosci 39(11):763–781, 2016

Sharon G, Sampson TR, Geschwind DH, et al: The central nervous system and the gut microbiome. Cell 167(4):915–932, 2016

Stetler C, Miller GE: Depression and hypothalamic-pituitary-adrenal activation: a quantitative summary of four decades of research. Psychosom Med 73(2):114–126, 2011

Szasz TS: The Myth of Mental Illness: Foundations of a Theory of Personal Conduct. New York, Harper & Row, 1961

Volkow ND, Fowler JS, Wang GJ, et al: Dopamine in drug abuse and addiction: results of imaging studies and treatment implications. Arch Neurol 64(11):1575–1579, 2007

Volkow ND, Fowler JS, Wang GJ, et al: Imaging dopamine's role in drug abuse and addiction. Neuropharmacology 56 (suppl 1):3–8, 2009

Waken RJ, De Las Fuentes L, Rao DC: A review of the genetics of hypertension with a focus on gene-environment interactions. Curr Hypertens Rep 19(3):23, 2017

Wise RA, Koob GF: The development and maintenance of drug addiction. Neuropsychopharmacology 39(2):254–262, 2014

Zhou L, Foster JA: Psychobiotics and the gut-brain axis: in the pursuit of happiness. Neuropsychiatr Dis Treat 11:715–723, 2015

Zorn JV, Schür RR, Boks MP, et al: Cortisol stress reactivity across psychiatric disorders: a systematic review and meta-analysis. Psychoneuroendocrinology 77:25–36, 2017

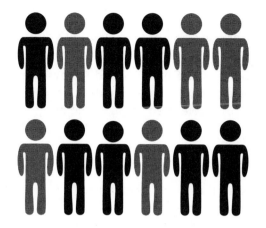

6

Mental Illness Is Serious

Half Truth: Mental illness is as bad as many physical illnesses.

Whole Truth: Mental illness is worse than most physical illnesses.

Important Points

- We fear medical illness because it causes death, disability, and deterioration.
- Compared with other medical illnesses, mental illness causes comparable levels of death, disability, and deterioration to those of other medical illnesses.
- Suicide is the second leading cause of death for people ages 10–35 years and the fourth leading cause of death for people ages 18–65 years.

- Mental illness is the number one cause of time lived with disability in the United States.
- Chronic mental illness shortens the lifespan and increases the risk of other medical illnesses such as diabetes and heart disease. Chronic mental illness causes accelerated aging of the body.

Introduction

Biological dysfunction is a necessary but not sufficient component of medical illness. Biological dysfunction alone does not indicate illness. As everyone intuitively knows, illness also entails suffering and disability. It does not take a physician to recognize the objective hallmarks of illness: Medical illness kills people, inhibits normal functioning, and causes physical deterioration. Although it is quite complicated to show that mental illnesses involve biological dysfunction, it is relatively easy to document disability, death, and comorbidity caused by mental illness. These data make our most powerful and important argument for the reality of mental illness, because what kills us is undeniably real.

This information also justifies the necessity of mental health treatment, making it the linchpin of effective advocacy. All medical treatments are inherently risky, and mental health treatments are both risky and controversial. Psychiatric medications may cause or contribute to diabetes, hypertension, cardiac arrhythmias, gastric ulcers, permanent neurological problems, and a host of other severe consequences. Other biological therapies such as electroconvulsive therapy have substantial risks as well. Even psychotherapy is expensive and time-consuming. It requires deep emotional vulnerability, and places people at risk for both emotional traumatization and exploitation from their therapists. Even after many months of psychotherapy, patients may have difficulty evaluating whether their therapy is working or whether the therapist should really be trusted.

The cost, time, and risk of psychiatric treatment can be justified in only one way: if treatment results in better outcomes than untreated illness. Put another way, if mental health disorders do not cause severe medical consequences, then mental health treatment is not justified. The accumulated consequences of moderate and severe mental illness are devastating, and even mild illness can impose a significant long-term burden on afflicted individuals. Mental illnesses are fully on par with other medical conditions in their ability to kill and disable people, and they substantially contribute to other chronic medical problems as well. These facts are easy to understand, and they make an irrefutable case for advocates: Mental illness is medically real, and the need for treatment is urgent.

Medical Illness: Why Do We Care?

When I was in medical training, I used to fantasize about getting sick. This is embarrassing to admit, but I envied some of the patients I saw in the hospital. Not all of them, of course. Some of them were in terrible pain or facing death. I felt terrible for anyone in that position, and I did not envy it. But I was exhausted, overworked, and under pressure, so I used to dream of being in the hospital for some correctable medical problem. That way, I could use sick days without using up my limited vacation time. No one could make me be on call or get up at 4 A.M. to go do patient rounds. People would bring me food or anything else I needed. I would not have any responsibility except to lie there and be taken care of. What if I needed something like gallbladder surgery, and then could lie in bed and recover for the next couple of weeks? Wouldn't that be great? Wouldn't it be like a vacation—or even better because no one would expect me to make up all the work I missed?

I now realize that being hospitalized would not be great. It would be bad. The hospital is a terrible place to relax, and even at home, being sick gets boring and tedious very quickly. It is never a vacation to be medically ill. Luckily for me, I did not get seriously ill in medical school. I did have a brush with illness during my psychiatry training, however. At about 4 A.M. one day, a strange, intense pain in my left lower back woke me up. It hurt enough to make me get up, move around, and see if I could work it out. I could not. It was too deep and steady for a muscle or joint pain, and it did not feel like a digestive problem. Whatever it was, it kept getting worse. I started to worry. What was wrong with me? It got so intense after about 15 minutes that I started to get dressed to go to the hospital. At this point, it became agonizing. I knew nothing but that intense, pure pain. At the same time, a little piece of my mind formed a bubble and started clicking through possible medical explanations. And because I had recently graduated from medical school, I quickly arrived at the worst possible diagnosis: a dissecting aortic aneurysm. I thought my aorta was about to explode and put my brief life to an end right there in front of the bedroom closet. I might not even make it to the hospital. I was genuinely petrified. Yet, weirdly enough, by the time I got to the emergency room, the pain was fading. By the time I saw the doctor, the pain was entirely gone. I felt like a fake, like the boy who cried wolf. I was so embarrassed that I celebrated openly when later told I had blood in my urine. I wasn't making this up! It turned out I had a kidney stone—a very painful condition, but hardly life-threatening. But it went on for weeks, causing me to be in and out of work, wondering where all of this was going to lead.

I tell these stories because they illustrate something about the experience of medical illness. When we are medically ill, seriously ill, we care somewhat about the biology of our illness. We care what the scans and lab tests say, and we care about the research on our illness. But we ultimately care for one reason: Medical illness is disrupting and threatening our lives. If medical illness did not do bad things to us, it would be only mildly interesting. It would not be overwhelmingly important to us as individuals or a society. If we want to look at how real and serious mental illness may be, we need to ask how often it does these bad things that illness can do.

What bad things does medical illness do? No one needs a textbook to answer this question, but for practical purposes we can divide them into three categories. The first one is death. This is very straightforward. I get seriously ill, and I wonder whether I will live or die. The second bad consequence of medical illness is disability. Maybe I won't die, but I wonder whether I will be able to work, or care for my family, or go out of my home and do things that are important in my life. Medical illness can disable me, even when it does not kill me. Finally, the third bad consequence is decline. Maybe this illness will not kill me or disable me, but what if my health deteriorates over time? What if I get weaker, less energetic, and more vulnerable to other illnesses? What if my health goes downhill and I die at a younger age, even if it is not from this particular illness? This can happen with quite a few chronic illnesses, including diabetes and high blood pressure. So the three dreadful consequences of medical illness are death, disability, and decline.

If we want to see whether mental illness is truly real, then we need to look at mental illness through the same lens as medical illness and see if it has the same consequences. No matter what the biology of mental illness may be, if mental illness is nothing more than a nuisance, if it is similar to having a bad mood or a bad day, then maybe it should not be in the same category as serious medical illnesses. Maybe people should just ignore the symptoms, toughen up, and go on. Maybe mental illness is physically real but does not have the same physical consequences as other illnesses. Sure, no one wants to feel anxious or depressed, but such a feeling is really not as bad as having cancer or heart disease, is it? Or is it? Can we really compare? Yes, we can compare. And in this chapter, we will use the same medical standards to compare the same medical consequences—death, disability, and decline—for mental and other medical illnesses.

Death

Sometimes our first instinct tells us that mental illness cannot really kill people. The symptoms are mental, so how can mental things like anxiety or hallucinations kill anyone? Maybe mental illness is like a bad dream. We all wake up from a bad dreams and breathe a sigh of relief, realizing the dream wasn't real and could not hurt us. "It was all in my head," we think. If people just realize their mental symptoms are "all in the head," then what is the harm?

Of course, must of us do not think this way for more than a few seconds before realizing that mental illness does, in fact, kill us. And there is one way that mental illness kills us very quickly and directly: suicide. Mental illnesses like depression can cause suicide, but so can other mental illnesses like substance abuse, anxiety, psychosis, and bipolar disorders. Careful studies over several decades have shown that around 90% of people in the U.S. who die by suicide have a mental illness (Bertolote et al. 2004; Cavanagh et al. 2003; Cho et al. 2016). So we can look at suicide rates and take them as a good estimate for people who die suddenly from mental illness. This is one way of seeing how often mental illness kills people compared with other medical illnesses. It is a way of comparing "apples to apples," using the same measures we use for other illnesses to see how real and severe mental illness may be.

Fortunately, suicide is quite rare among children. Sadly, as shown in Table 6–1, suicide is the number two medical cause of death for teenagers, and remains the second highest cause for individuals into the mid-30s. Only accidents cause more deaths in these age groups. Considering that substance use is involved in more than 50% of motor vehicle fatalities, it seems likely that some of those accidents are also due to mental illness (Brady and Li 2014).

In individuals ages 35–54 years, suicide is the fourth-highest medical cause of death. After that (ages 55–64), suicide falls to eight, and finally out of the top 10 for people 65 and older. But this does not mean that people over age 65 die less often by suicide. Suicide kills just as many people in old age as in other times of life. Yet other causes of death become more common by comparison, pushing suicide down the "charts." At the same time, Alzheimer's dementia is the number five cause of death for people over age 65, and Alzheimer's dementia is a mental illness. So mental illness is in the top 10 medical causes of death for every age group over 9 years old (Centers for Disease Control and Prevention 2017) (Table 6–2).

For people in their prime adult years, ages 18–65, suicide and mental illness are listed fourth among the medical causes of death (Table 6–3). Suicide and mental illness kill more people in this age group than diabetes, HIV, strokes, liver disease, or lung disease. In fact, suicide kills more people than homicide—a lot more. Suicide and mental illness kill more than twice as many people every year than murder in this age group, and more than three times as many people of all ages (Centers for Disease Control and Prevention 2020). You

TABLE 6–1.   Top 10 medical causes of death in the United States
in 2017, ages 10–30 years

AGES 10–30 YEARS	
1. Accident (29,529)	6. Congenital abnormalities (803)
2. Suicide (11,577)	7. Diabetes mellitus (703)
3. Homicide (8,680)	8. Cerebrovascular disease (485)
4. Cancer (3,462)	9. Complicated pregnancy (475)
5. Heart disease (2,628)	10. Chronic lung disease (441)

Source.   Adapted from Centers for Disease Control and Prevention 2017.

are more than three times as likely to kill yourself than to be killed by anyone else. Incidentally, many people fear being killed by a stranger with psychotic mental illness, but studies show that the odds of being killed by a
stranger with psychotic mental illness are unimaginably small—1 in 14.7
million or 0.000007% per year (Nielssen et al. 2009). So you are 1,820 times
more likely to die by suicide than to be killed by a stranger with psychosis!
In fact, people with mental illness are more likely to be the victims of violence than to inflict it on others. People with mental illness suffer four times
as much violence as the average person (Hughes et al. 2012).

How real is mental illness? Mental illness is real enough to kill you, and
kill you more often than most other kinds of illness. If we combine suicide
and Alzheimer's disease to calculate deaths by mental illness, we find that
mental illness ranks as the number four cause of death in our country for
all age groups combined (Centers for Disease Control and Prevention
2020). And rates of suicide are going up in this country, by an astounding
30% since 1999 (Stone et al. 2018). If all of this does not get our attention,
maybe we should wonder if we are in a state of denial about the realities of
these ravaging diseases.

Before moving on to discuss disability, I would like to say a couple of additional things about suicide. First, I can never think about this topic without feeling pain, both for people who died by suicide and for their loved
ones. People I love have died by suicide, and I know that pain. The grief that
follows the loss of someone to suicide is unlike any other grief. Suicide causes
a unique shame and ravaging guilt for people left behind. When people are
suicidal, they almost always think, "I'm just making it worse for everyone
around me. They will be sad for a while after I die, but then they will be
happier without me." No, they will not. I have never met a single person
who was remotely happy about having lost someone to suicide. I once sat

TABLE 6–2.   Top 10 medical causes of death in the United States, ages 1–85+

AGES 1–85+ YEARS

1. Heart disease (647,113)	6. Alzheimer's disease (121,402)
2. Cancer (599,042)	7. Diabetes mellitus (83,562)
3. Accident (168,603)	8. Influenza + pneumonia (55,514)
4. Chronic lung disease (160,179)	9. Nephritis (50,554)
5. Cerebrovascular disease (146,281)	**10. Suicide (47,168)**

Source.   Adapted from Centers for Disease Control and Prevention 2017.

in a hospital room with an 84-year-old man who was sobbing and still depressed over the suicide of his father when he (the son) was 14. Suicide is so common, and the pain is so great, that I never want to pass by the subject without acknowledging the wounds so many people bear from it.

Second, I think we need to consider whether all these data about suicide accurately reflect mental illness as a cause. One report is that 54% of people who die by suicide have a diagnosed mental illness (Stone et al. 2018). This report comes from data collected from 27 of the 50 states by the Centers for Disease Control and Prevention (CDC). It is good data, but it is often misinterpreted. It would be natural for someone to look at this number and think that 46% of people who die by suicide do not have a mental illness. But this is not the case. It turns out that only about 40% of people with mental illness have received any kind of treatment in the past year (Kessler et al. 2005). Therefore, it might not be surprising that around the same number of those who die by suicide do not have a *diagnosed* mental health condition. The CDC's data are from coroners' and law enforcement reports; therefore, these data tell us that at least 56% of people who die by suicide had a diagnosed mental illness, but they tell us nothing about the other 44%. And this is not an unusual situation, medically speaking. In medical school, I was told that the first sign of heart disease is sudden death in 50% of cases—in other words, a large proportion of people who die of heart disease have never been diagnosed, and the same applies for mental illness. Because of this, we look to more detailed studies of suicide, which give us a 90% figure (discussed in second paragraph of this section). Meanwhile, the CDC wants the public to know that we should not assume there is no risk of suicide among people who might not have a mental illness; there are other important factors in suicide, such as substance intoxication and loss of a relationship (Stone et al. 2018).

TABLE 6–3. Top 10 medical causes of death in the United States in 2017, ages 18–65

AGES 18–65	
1. Cancer (184,943)	6. Chronic lung disease (26,683)
2. Heart disease (137,677)	7. Diabetes mellitus (26,349)
3. Accident (110,001)	8. Cerebrovascular disease (22,202)
4. **Suicide (37,380)**	9. Homicide (16,939)
5. Liver disease (27,175)	10. Septicemia (blood infection) (10,394)

Source. Adapted from Centers for Disease Control and Prevention 2017.

Disability

If mental illness is deadly, is it also disabling? And how often does it disable people compared with other medical illnesses? If you have been reading this book carefully, you will not be surprised by the answer: number one. Mental illness is the number one cause of years lived with disability (YLDs) in this country (Figure 6–1). That is to say, as a group mental illnesses cause more time spent in disability than joint diseases (like arthritis), lung diseases (like emphysema), or even heart disease (Murray et al. 2013; Mokdad et al. 2018). And among single illnesses, major depression is the number two cause of years lived with disability in this country, and number one in the world (Mokdad et al. 2018; Ferrari et al. 2013; World Health Organization 2017). Nine of the top 25 medical causes of disability (in YLDs) are mental illnesses (Mokdad et al. 2018). And while time in disability is only one way of measuring medical disability, various measures of disability always find mental illnesses among the top causes. For instance, when researchers combine years *lived* in disability with years *lost* to disability (due to premature death), mental illnesses still account for 6 of the top 25 medical causes of "disability-adjusted life years" (DALYs) (Mokdad et al. 2018). Mental illnesses are profoundly disabling.

Many who encounter these numbers will be tempted to scoff. When some people hear of disability, they think of those who do not want to work, or people "faking it for a disability check." While this reaction is understandable, it is wrong. Of course, some people may fake mental illness, as they may fake back pain and other medical conditions, but mental illness is still the leading cause of disability. How do we know? Because mental illness

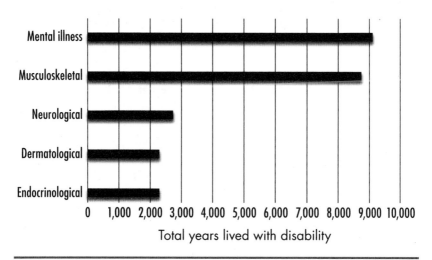

FIGURE 6–1. Medical illnesses and years of life lived with disability. As a category of medical illness, mental illness accounted for more years lived with disability (YLDs) than any other category of medical illness in the United States in 2016. YLDs are one important medical measurement of disability.
Source. Data from Mokdad et al. 2018.

is a top cause of disability in countries all over the world, even in countries that do not have disability payments or even mental health systems. In fact, mental illness accounts for about one-third of time lost to disability worldwide, and mental illnesses make up 5 of the top 20 disabling illnesses in the world (Vigo et al. 2016). These numbers are comparable to those found in the United States (Merikangas et al. 2007). Mental illness is profoundly disabling, regardless of whether people have support or not. I know this from personal experience, as I see the anguish of people with mental illness who try repeatedly to work but simply cannot function enough to do so. They hardly consider their situation to be a vacation. Instead, they struggle with feelings of guilt, worthlessness, and hopelessness. People with mental illness are normal people who have mental illness. They want the same things that everyone else wants, and they want to be productive, contributing people who feel good about their work—just like everyone else.

Decline

Even when illness does not kill or disable us, it can take a toll on our physical health. Chronic illness creates wear and tear on the body, making us weaker, less energetic, and more prone to other illnesses. In the end, chronic illness can cause us to live shorter lives, and spend the time we have in a state of worsened health. Diabetes is a well-known example of this problem: Even with treatment, diabetes can shorten life, impair people's physical abilities over time, and make them vulnerable to kidney problems, infection, and heart disease. Diabetes is a common reason that people need limb amputations or dialysis for kidney disease.

Can mental illness do the same thing? At first glance, it seems un-likely—so unlikely that for many decades no one really tried to answer the question. However, there is now mounting evidence that mental illness takes a toll on the body, just as other chronic medical illnesses do. One review of over 90 studies involving 1.7 million people showed that mental illnesses shorten the lifespan by an average of 10 years. These illnesses include anx-iety, depression, bipolar disorder, and schizophrenia (Chesney et al. 2014). Increased substance use problems are major causes of premature death and have lowered the average life expectancy for the entire population in recent years (Rehm and Probst 2018). Overall, compared with the general popu-lation, people with a mental illness are twice as likely to die in any given pe-riod of time (Walker et al. 2015). This is an extraordinary increase, and it is even worse for more severe cases of mental illness. For instance, those with schizophrenia have about triple the risk of death in any given time pe-riod (Olfson et al. 2015).

The vast majority of these deaths are not due to suicide. Instead, people with mental illness are more likely to die of heart disease, stroke, infection, and accidents. They are also more likely to die of cancer, although they may be no more likely to get cancer in the first place (Kisely et al. 2013). Mental illnesses are significant risk factors for a variety of other serious illnesses. Anxiety disorders increase the risk of stroke by 24% (Perez-Pinar et al. 2016). People with severe mental illness such as schizophrenia and bipolar disorder are two to three times more likely to die of cardiovascular disease (Liu et al. 2017). Depression is also bad for the heart, both emotionally and physically. Among people who have had a heart attack, having depression doubles the risk of having another. This risk is similar to the effects of diabe-tes on heart disease (Cohen et al. 2015). Major depression increases the risk of getting heart disease in the first place, and it also increases the risk of get-ting diabetes by about 40% (Rotella and Mannucci 2013). Schizophrenia and bipolar disorder are accompanied by worse control of blood sugar, and thereby also increase the risk for diabetes (Vancampfort et al. 2016). Over-all, mental illnesses account for an estimated 14% of all deaths worldwide (Walker et al. 2015).

Why are mental illnesses so hard on the body? I have already discussed some of the reasons: Mental illnesses disrupt hormones, alter digestion and gut bacteria, and ramp up the inflammatory system (see Chapter 5). The resultant chronic physical stress takes a toll on the body over time and puts it at risk for many other diseases. Looking at these data, scientists have begun to put together ways in which chronic mental illness speeds up the aging process. One example is posttraumatic stress disorder (PTSD). Like many other mental illnesses, PTSD causes people to die younger and to get more illnesses of old age (such as dementia and heart disease) at a younger age. But PTSD also increases some other biological markers of old age, such as inflammation. One of the most interesting is called telomere length. *Telomere* is just a name for the end of a chromosome (string of DNA). When a cell divides, the telomere gets shorter, so telomeres are a good marker for aging of cells. Shorter telomeres mean older cells, and it turns out that telomeres are shorter in PTSD (Lohr et al. 2015). The same is true for depression, anxiety, and schizophrenia (Vakonaki et al. 2018). In fact, many mental illnesses appear to accelerate aging in a variety of ways. Researchers have found this to be the case with bipolar disorder, schizophrenia, and depression (Kirkpatrick et al. 2007; Koutsouleris et al. 2013; Wolkowitz et al. 2011).

The Reality of Mental Illness: Walking the Walk

Mental illness is serious business. It kills; it disables; it wears down bodies and brains. It increases risk for heart disease and diabetes. It makes people age faster. Is mental illness as bad as most other kinds of medical illnesses? No. Mental illness is worse than most other kinds of medical illnesses. Mental illness accounts for more deaths, more disability, and more poor health than most other kinds of medical illness. And we can see that clearly when we treat mental illness as we do any other form of medical illness, by applying the same standards of measurement that we use with other medical illnesses. Mental illness is real, and it is bad.

In one sense, such findings come as a relief for those of us who experience mental illness: We are not faking. We are not making it seem worse than it is. We are not being lazy or irresponsible. And we are not being weak when we ask for medical treatment of mental illness. We are being responsible, just as we have to be responsible when we get other forms of illness. If the illness is severe, we need to stay home, rest, recover, take care of ourselves, seek treatment, and follow doctors' advice. We do not need to listen to all the well-meaning people who say to us, "Stop feeling sorry for yourself," or "Just get up and focus on other people," or (even worse) "Stop making yourself sick."

By the way, this is a good reminder for all of us about how *not* to act when we encounter people with mental illness. We should treat people with mental illness just as we want to treat people with other medical illnesses. We should not look down on them for having an illness, and we should not start lecturing them about what to do. What if you visited an emergency room to see a friend right after a heart attack? Would you say, "I think we might as well admit that you brought this on yourself. It's time for you to take some responsibility, stop feeling sorry for yourself, and get on with your life. It's not all about you, you know"? And yet people have been told such things in emergency rooms right after suicide attempts. In the past, even medical professionals have been unsympathetic or judgmental to those who have nearly died by suicide.

Consider whether you would go up to someone with cancer and suggest, "You know, I'd get off that chemotherapy you are using. I read online that it's got some bad side effects, and it's probably just making you worse. Maybe you don't even have cancer in the first place. Why don't you stop depending on some pill and live in a healthy way instead?" No one would say that to a cancer patient, and yet many people with mental illness are advised to get off their medicines or try other treatments by people who are neither medical professionals nor family members. Some are even told they are not sick. So we should remember not to play doctor when someone we love has mental illness. I am a doctor myself, but when I am not officially someone's doctor, I do not try to be a doctor to that person. I try to be a good friend, or family member, or coworker.

How *should* we act toward individuals suffering from episodes of mental illness? The same way we act toward those suffering from any illness. We might send a card, tell them we are thinking of them, bake them some cookies, offer a ride to an appointment, or ask if they need anything. We might remember that they are sick, and not wait for them to reach out to us. We need to respect the privacy of those with mental illness, but not to the point of ignoring them. Most of all, we need to listen to what they tell us when we do reach out. We must listen and respond sensitively, just as we would for any other kind of illness.

On one hand, the medical reality of mental illness helps us to support those who have it, and it helps us to avoid guilt and shame when we have it ourselves. It is a relief, an affirmation that those who suffer are not inferior or at fault. On the other hand, mental illness is terrifyingly destructive. If you have a mental illness, you are likely to experience quite a few unsettling questions: Will I die earlier? Will I get other diseases too? Is my body falling apart as we speak?

The answer is that we are not doomed. The rest of this book contains some of the good news about mental illness, but I want to say right now that the subject of mental illness should not be depressing to us as we look to the future. We should feel inspired. For the first time in human history, we *know*, scientifically, that mental illnesses *are* real medical illnesses. And for the first time in human history, we have real, scientifically tested treatments for mental illnesses. The situation is not hopeless, and it gets more hopeful every day.

We will talk more about treatment in Chapter 7, but let me give a few examples here to show that we are not doomed. Yes, mental illness speeds up cellular aging (shortened telomeres), but did you know that some treatments for mental illness activate an enzyme than lengthens telomeres (Bersani et al. 2015)? Mental illnesses cause neurons to shrivel and die, but many psychiatric treatments (including medications) and other factors (such as exercise) increase the birth and growth of neurons (Baek 2016; Hunsberger et al. 2009). We can indeed see abnormal brain activity on head scans, but both psychotherapy (talk therapy) and psychiatric medications have been shown to change those patterns in other head scan studies (Barsaglini et al. 2014).

Mental illness is a powerful risk factor for death, disability, and decline, but it is only one risk factor among others. For example, you may have mental illness and run the risk of diabetes, but maybe diabetes does not run in your family (genetic factors). Even if it does, you can make a bigger impact by changing your diet and exercising (lifestyle factors). One of the biggest factors in long-term health is controlling your stress level, and we have many good ways of doing that. Even things such as social support (connections to other people) and spirituality have been shown to lessen inflammation, improve overall health, and lengthen life (Shattuck and Muehlenbein 2020; Uchino et al. 2018). In other words, no one is doomed. We have more tools today to deal with mental illness than ever before, and we will have still greater resources in days to come.

Is Mental Illness Real: Why All the Controversy?

I suspect that anyone reading about the medical reality of mental illness and then rereading Chapter 4 on the controversies about mental illness would feel a bit confused. On the one hand, the evidence is in: Thousands and thousands of studies tell us that mental illness is real biological illness with real medical consequences. On the other hand, there are still controversies about whether mental illness is merely a cultural construct, whether mental illnesses are just made up, and whether medical treatment of mental illness is a bad thing. If the science is so clear, then why all the controversy?

Mental Illness: Mental vs. Physical

I can think of two reasons why controversy remains, although there are probably many more. The first reason is cultural: Our culture is gradually but fitfully accepting the idea that something can be both mental and physical at the same time. When I was growing up in the 1960s and 1970s, everyone intuitively knew that things had to be either physical or mental. Mental might mean intellectual, or spiritual, or even emotional, but mental certainly did not mean physical. Bodies could break down and physically sicken, but minds and spirits could not. So everyone I knew was fine with the idea that if someone has a physical problem like diabetes, the person should take a physical medicine like insulin. When it came to mental problems, things got complicated. Intuitively, we all felt as if thoughts, feelings, and behaviors were things we should control. Of course, people did get out of hand at times, losing their temper or fighting or getting washed away in sadness, but they were told to "get a hold of themselves," to "pull themselves together." We all expected ourselves to exert self-control, to "shape up or ship out." It was a matter of shame, of personal and moral failure, when we did lose control. If mental problems were not physical, then they had to be mental. And if they were mental, then taking a physical medicine for them, or even seeing a doctor, did not make sense. Seeking physical treatment for mental problems sounded like a mistake. More than that, it seemed like a morally bad idea, a personal failure. So people were doubtful and ashamed about seeking medical treatment for mental problems.

What changed? The science changed, and a revolution in neuroscience occurred. Today, we know differently. We know that mental events—thoughts, feelings, and behaviors—are both mental and physical. And because mental life is also physical, it is subject to physical illness. To the extent that mental illness is physical, it ought to be treated physically and medically. Yet human beings still show a tendency to separate the physical from the mental (Bloom 2004), and old ways of thinking die hard (Ahn et al. 2006). Cultural change tends to occur gradually over generations, so many people still have a vague feeling that there is something morally wrong with psychiatry and mental health treatment.

The second reason is scientific: We still do not completely understand mental illnesses. We do not yet have all the biology figured out. We know more than enough to know that mental illness is physical, but we do not know enough to know just how each mental illness works. We treat mental illnesses with medications and hospitalization, yet we do not fully understand what we are treating. How can this be? Because most mental illnesses are syndromes, and not diseases. This is a statement that sounds strange and deserves some explanation. I think you will find it worth your time to understand the distinction, because it helps us understand much of the controversy about mental illness.

Mental Illness: Syndromes vs. Diseases

What is a syndrome? *Syndrome* is a medical term for a collection of signs and symptoms. *Signs* are things a doctor can see objectively, and *symptoms* are things that a patient reports. You tell your doctor symptoms, and then the doctor examines you for signs of illness. Together, a set of signs and symptoms makes up a syndrome. But one syndrome can have many different medical causes. For instance, having a cold (an upper respiratory infection) is a syndrome. A person can have symptoms such as a sore throat, nasal congestion, achiness, and fatigue, and signs such as fever, cough, and a red, inflamed throat. Yet many different things can cause a cold. There are many different viruses that can do so. Bacteria can do so—strep throat is one example of cold symptoms from bacterial infection. Even allergies can sometimes make people feel that they have a cold, though we can usually tell the difference between the two. So the cold is a syndrome and indicates an illness, although it can have different causes. Many people never think about illnesses this way, but pneumonia is a syndrome with different causes, and so is high blood pressure. Every syndrome is the same way: one condition that can have several different causes.

When we can match a syndrome to the underlying cause, then we call it a *disease* (Figure 6–2). For instance, strep throat is a disease, because we can match the syndrome (upper respiratory illness) to the underlying cause (infection by streptococcal bacteria). A syndrome like upper respiratory infection is still a real illness, even when we do not know the cause. When we can diagnose the precise cause (such as streptococcal bacterial infection), then we call it a disease.

Depression is another medical syndrome that has many causes. For instance, underactive thyroid (hypothyroidism), Vitamin D deficiency, and quite a few other medical problems can cause depression. More than a few medicines can give people depression, and lots of people have gotten depressed by drinking too much alcohol. Yet we do not know the underlying disease for most cases of major depression. There may, in fact, be hundreds of different underlying causes still to be discovered. And this is likely to be true of most mental illnesses. There may turn out to be, for instance, 20 different kinds of autism, 30 different kinds of schizophrenia, and 40 different kinds of anxiety. We know that all of those are biological illnesses, just as we know that a cold is a biological illness. But we do not know all the underlying causes, so right now our research and diagnosis focus on syndromes.

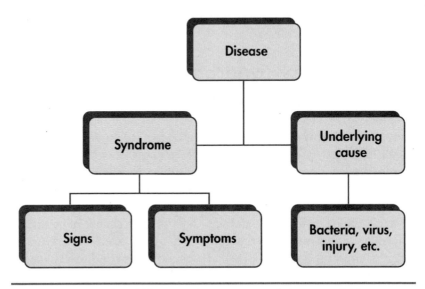

FIGURE 6–2. The difference between syndromes and diseases.
A syndrome is a common collection of medical signs and symptoms. Syndromes can have a variety of underlying causes. When we know the underlying cause of a syndrome, we can diagnose a disease.

This uncertainty about the underlying causes of mental illness should not alarm anyone. In every branch of medicine, we do not know all the causes for all the syndromes we treat. We do not always know what is causing high blood pressure, but we can still treat it medically. The same applies for migraine headaches, but nobody doubts the reality of migraine headaches, and doctors do not hesitate to prescribe medicines for them. Many autoimmune disorders have unknown causes, but they are still frighteningly real. Because the brain is so complex, it is no surprise that we will need a lot more research to define all of the underlying diseases. But we do not need research for us to know with confidence that mental illness is real medical illness, any more than we need research to know that pneumonia is real medical illness.

I believe this uncertainty is the source of most controversy about mental illnesses today. Psychiatrists do get together in committees to vote on what qualifies as a mental illness in DSM. However, they do not simply make up illnesses. Instead, they look and see what constitutes a clear medical syndrome (a clear collection of signs and symptoms) supported by evidence that it is medically real (biological dysfunction with health consequences). Countless studies go into these decisions, and both the general public and other mental health professionals are invited to give feedback. There is nothing secretive or arbitrary about the decisions involved.

Why do professionals go to this trouble? Why do they bother defining precise medical syndromes? There are two reasons: diagnosis and research. If everyone can agree about the definition of these illnesses (syndromes), then people with the same problems can be diagnosed in the same way. Once individuals have been diagnosed, they need treatments. Agreement about these illnesses means that we have proven treatments for specific syndromes. For example, we have thousands of studies on treating major depression, and these guide doctors and other mental health professionals in applying scientific treatments. They also guide researchers in discovering treatments for these carefully defined syndromes. Thus, doctors and researchers are all working with the same idea of what it means to diagnose and treat illnesses such as schizophrenia and obsessive-compulsive disorder.

Finally, understanding that we are working with syndromes helps explain why mental health treatment today is powerful but not precise. When someone is diagnosed with a syndrome such as schizophrenia or bipolar disorder, we have powerful treatments to offer. Yet we do not know precisely which treatments (especially which combination of medicines and psychotherapy) will be effective for each particular person. Each person is biologically different, and each syndrome may have many different causes. Therefore, we can offer a medicine that will work for most people with the syndrome, without being sure whether this medicine is the best one for this particular individual.

This treatment dilemma is common in medical practice. Most people take an antibiotic after the doctor has made a guess about the cause of a particular syndrome (such as ear infection or sinus infection). In most cases, doctors make an educated guess about which antibiotic will work best, without knowing which bacteria is behind the infection, or without being positive that there is a bacterial infection. If the patient does not respond, the doctor can change the antibiotic or do further testing.

The same is true for treating mental health conditions. We try a medicine that is likely to work, but if it doesn't, we change the medicine or reevaluate the medical situation. In some ways, this is making a guess, but it is a highly educated and thoughtful guess, backed up by solid science. Most people eventually get partial or full relief of their symptoms, but unfortunately they have to be persistent, just like people getting treatment for diabetes or high blood pressure. The first medication does not always work, and usually medication should be combined with other interventions, such as diet and exercise, in order to be completely successful.

In the future, we will not have to settle for highly educated guessing. We will get lab tests and a head scan and know with precision which treatments will work best. This *will* happen, because it is already starting to happen. Although this process is just beginning in psychiatry, it is well advanced in some specialties such as oncology. People with some types of cancer can undergo genetic testing for themselves and their cancer, and often know precisely which treatments will work best. This type of treatment will revolutionize medical treatment in most specialties, including psychiatry. It is only a matter of time.

Meanwhile, the situation now is not as dire as most people think. Not knowing everything does not mean that we don't know anything. We know a lot, and we don't know a lot. We know mental illness is real, and we know our treatments are real. But we have so far to go, so much distance between complete ignorance and complete truth. We find ourselves in between the two, in an exciting but exasperating time in the history of brain science. New and exciting advances occur nearly every day, but it takes years and decades to answer the most important questions and get the lifesaving treatments we need. The situation is immeasurably better than it was 50 years ago, but not nearly as good as it will be in 50 more years. Meanwhile, people with mental illness need relief now. So let's move on to some relief and discuss some of the good news about mental illness.

Advice for Advocacy

- Data demonstrating the medical seriousness of mental illness is the most central and powerful evidence we have for advocacy.
- But it need not be the longest or most complex part of the discussion. These data allow us to present in a simple and straightforward manner: Mental illness kills us, disables us, and undermines our health.
- Comparisons with other types of medical illness are more powerful than raw data alone. Numbers need context: Forty thousand people may die of suicide every year in the United States. This is an overwhelming number, but what does it mean in a country of 330 million people?
- Remember that suicide is an especially sensitive topic for many. Whenever we discuss suicide, we need to show empathy for those who have lost people to suicide.
- Data about medical consequences of mental illness may be especially powerful, but it may be particularly discouraging to those who have mental illness. They may wonder whether they are doomed to be destroyed by their illness. So some reassurance

with hopeful information is important when dealing with this material.

- Understanding the difference between syndromes and diseases is critically important for mental health professionals, and important for understanding the nature of DSM. But it will often be more relevant in medical or academic settings than in advocacy with the general public.

References

Ahn WK, Flanagan EH, Marsh JK, et al: Beliefs about essences and the reality of mental disorders. Psychol Sci 17(9):759–766, 2006

Baek SS: Role of exercise on the brain. J Exerc Rehabil 12(5):380–385, 2016

Barsaglini A, Sartori G, Benetti S, et al: The effects of psychotherapy on brain function: a systematic and critical review. Prog Neurobiol 114:1–14, 2014

Bersani FS, Lindqvist D, Mellon SH, et al: Telomerase activation as a possible mechanism of action for psychopharmacological interventions. Drug Discov Today 20(11):1305–1309, 2015

Bertolote JM, Fleischmann A, De Leo D, et al: Psychiatric diagnoses and suicide: revisiting the evidence. Crisis 25(4):147–155, 2004

Bloom P: Descartes' Baby: How the Science of Child Development Explains What Makes Us Human. New York, Basic Books, 2004

Brady JE, Li G: Trends in alcohol and other drugs detected in fatally injured drivers in the United States, 1999–2010. Am J Epidemiol 179(6):692–699, 2014

Cavanagh JT, Carson AJ, Sharpe M, et al: Psychological autopsy studies of suicide: a systematic review. Psychol Med 33(3):395–405, 2003

Centers for Disease Control and Prevention: 10 Leading Causes of Death by Age Group—2017. National Vital Statistic System, National Center for Health Statistics, CDC, 2017. Available at: www.cdc.gov/injury/wisqars/pdf/leading_causes_of_death_by_age_group_2017-508.pdf. Accessed July 30, 2020.

Centers for Disease Control and Prevention: Ten Leading Causes of Death and Injury. National Center for Injury Prevention and Control, March 20, 2020. Available at: www.cdc.gov/injury/wisqars/LeadingCauses.html. Accessed July 30, 2020.

Chesney E, Goodwin GM, Fazel S: Risks of all-cause and suicide mortality in mental disorders: a meta-review. World Psychiatry 13(2):153–160, 2014

Cho SE, Na KS, Cho SJ, et al: Geographical and temporal variations in the prevalence of mental disorders in suicide: systematic review and meta-analysis. J Affect Disord 190:704–713, 2016

Cohen BE, Edmondson D, Kronish IM: State of the art review: depression, stress, anxiety, and cardiovascular disease. Am J Hypertens 28(11):1295–1302, 2015

Ferrari AJ, Charlson FJ, Norman RE, et al: Burden of depressive disorders by country, sex, age, and year: findings from the global burden of disease study 2010. PLoS Med 10(11):e1001547, 2013

114   Science Over Stigma

Hughes K, Bellis MA, Jones L, et al: Prevalence and risk of violence against adults with disabilities: a systematic review and meta-analysis of observational studies. Lancet 379(9826):1621–1629, 2012
Hunsberger J, Austin DR, Henter ID, et al: The neurotrophic and neuroprotective effects of psychotropic agents. Dialogues Clin Neurosci 11(3):333–348, 2009
Kessler RC, Chiu WT, Demler O, et al: Prevalence, severity, and comorbidity of 12-month DSM-IV disorders in the national comorbidity survey replication. Arch Gen Psychiatry 62(6):617–627, 2005
Kirkpatrick B, Messias E, Harvey PD, et al: Is schizophrenia a syndrome of accelerated aging? Schizophr Bull 34(6):1024–1032, 2007
Kisely S, Crowe E, Lawrence D: Cancer-related mortality in people with mental illness. JAMA Psychiatry 70(2):209–217, 2013
Koutsouleris N, Davatzikos C, Borgwardt S, et al: Accelerated brain aging in schizophrenia and beyond: a neuroanatomical marker of psychiatric disorders. Schizophr Bull 40(5):1140–1153, 2013
Liu NH, Daumit GL, Dua T, et al: Excess mortality in persons with severe mental disorders: a multilevel intervention framework and priorities for clinical practice, policy and research agendas. World Psychiatry 16(1):30–40, 2017
Lohr JB, Palmer BW, Eidt CA, et al: Is post-traumatic stress disorder associated with premature senescence? A review of the literature. Am J Geriatr Psychiatry 23(7):709–725, 2015
Merikangas KR, Ames M, Cui L, et al: The impact of comorbidity of mental and physical conditions on role disability in the U.S. adult household population. Arch Gen Psychiatry 64(10):1180–1188, 2007
Mokdad AH, Ballestros K, Echko M, et al: The state of U.S. health, 1990–2016: burden of diseases, injuries, and risk factors among U.S. states. JAMA 319(14):1444–1472, 2018
Murray CJ, Abraham J, Ali MK, et al: The state of U.S. health, 1990–2010: burden of diseases, injuries, and risk factors. JAMA 310(6):591–606, 2013
Nielssen O, Bourget D, Laajasalo T, et al: Homicide of strangers by people with a psychotic illness. Schizophr Bull 37(3):572–579, 2009
Olfson M, Gerhard T, Huang C, et al: Premature mortality among adults with schizophrenia in the United States. JAMA Psychiatry 72(12):1172–1181, 2015
Perez-Pinar M, Ayerbe L, González E, et al: Anxiety disorders and risk of stroke: a systematic review and meta-analysis. Eur Psychiatry 41:102–108, 2016
Rehm J, Probst C: Decreases of life expectancy despite decreases in non-communicable disease mortality: the role of substance use and socioeconomic status. Eur Addict Res 24(2):53–59, 2018
Rotella F, Mannucci E: Depression as a risk factor for diabetes: a meta-analysis of longitudinal studies. J Clin Psychiatry 74(1):31–37, 2013
Shattuck EC, Muehlenbein MP: Religiosity/spirituality and physiological markers of health. J Relig Health 59(2):1035–1054, 2020
Stone DM, Simon TR, Fowler KA, et al: Vital signs: Trends in state suicide rates—United States, 1999–2016 and circumstances contributing to suicide—27 states, 2015. MMWR Morb Mortal Wkly Rep 67(22):617–624, 2018
Uchino BN, Bowen K, de Grey RK, et al: Social support and physical health: models, mechanisms, and opportunities, in Principles and Concepts of Behavioral Medicine. New York, Springer, 2018, pp 341–372

Vakonaki E, Tsiminikaki K, Plaitis S, et al: Common mental disorders and association with telomere length. Biomed Rep 8(2):111–116, 2018

Vancampfort D, Correll CU, Galling B, et al: Diabetes mellitus in people with schizophrenia, bipolar disorder and major depressive disorder: a systematic review and large scale meta-analysis. World Psychiatry 15(2):166–174, 2016

Vigo D, Thornicroft G, Atun R: Estimating the true global burden of mental illness. Lancet Psychiatry 3(2):171–178, 2016

Walker ER, McGee RE, Druss BG: Mortality in mental disorders and global disease burden implications: a systematic review and meta-analysis. JAMA Psychiatry 72(4):334–341, 2015

Wolkowitz OM, Reus VI, Mellon SH: Of sound mind and body: depression, disease, and accelerated aging. Dialogues Clin Neurosci 13(1):25–39, 2011

World Health Organization: Depression and Other Common Mental Disorders: Global Health Estimates. Geneva, World Health Organization, 2017

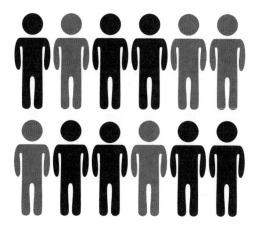

Mental Illness Is Nobody's Fault

Half Truth: Bad parenting, bad decisions, and bad habits all contribute to mental illness.

Whole Truth: Everyone has experienced bad parenting, bad habits, and bad decisions, but only some get mental illness, because of genes plus stress.

Important Points

- Parents have been wrongly and destructively blamed for mentally illness—most notably the "schizophrenogenic mother."
- "Toxic psychiatrists" have been blamed for mental illness, allegedly overdiagnosing and overtreating something that does not exist.
- Most of all, people with mental illness have been wrongly and destructively blamed for having it.

- The real cause of mental illness is not "psychiatrists plus parents plus patients," but genes plus stress.
- No one picks their genes, and no one picks their stresses in life, so no one is to blame for mental illness.
- Bad habits do contribute to illness, but everyone has bad habits. So the people who get sick from them are no different from those who do not get sick.

Introduction

Blame, shame, and guilt have always been the grim fellow travelers of mental illness. Every clinician can testify to the fact that these feelings whisper in the ears of patients and their families, contributing to denial, treatment avoidance, despair, and suicide. At least we now have the science to show that mental health disorders can never constitute subhuman inferiority, character flaws, or demonic influence. However, proving to the public that mental illnesses are legitimate medical illnesses is not enough to end stigma. Mental health professionals and their allies have successfully negotiated this fundamental challenge, convincing the public and governments that at least the major mental illnesses are biological disorders. This alone is a titanic accomplishment, one fundamental to our undertaking. Yet studies show that grasping this information does not eliminate all social stigma against mental illness (Mannarini and Rossi 2019). We will also need to address fears of dangerousness, visceral prejudice against social nonconformity, and wariness of the poverty that so often accompanies these disorders.

More fundamentally, most patients and families I know still struggle with residual guilt and shame, even when it cuts against their intellectual understanding of mental health problems. I can personally testify to this experience as a close family member of several people with mental illness. I will never forget one "family weekend" at an addiction treatment center, one I had contemplated with dismal dread during the preceding weeks. I knew I would attend, both because of familial love and because I could not live with the shame of skipping the event. Yet I badly wanted to miss it. As a parent, I had been over my own mistakes countless times, ingeniously connecting them to the problems of family members. I knew that other parents might feel the same guilt, but knew also that their faults were excusable. Other parents were not mental health professionals, and so could be excused for contributing to their children's problems. I, on the other hand, had no such excuse. I was a supposed expert in mental illness, and yet felt I had failed dismally as a parent. I knew I was substantially to blame.

I journeyed to the center with the sick feeling of a child marching to the principal's office. Yet much of the weekend proved anticlimactic. I somehow expected more dramatic intensity directed toward myself (as a parent) than I had ever witnessed (as a clinician) in any other treatment setting. But the approach here was gentle, uninvasive, and frankly elementary. It was only after a few hours of benumbed boredom that I began to consider what I was hearing: The addiction and the other illnesses were not my fault! I had heard this repeatedly during the day but had not listened because I "already knew it." I knew it intellectually but had not exposed myself emotionally, so the knowledge covered my personal guilt and shame like a hard candy coating. After a few minutes of befuddled insight, I finally felt the shock and relief—this truth actually did apply to me and to my guilt, when (like everyone else) I had considered myself a lone exception. This was such an elementary realization and such a liberating moment. In such simple moments, true healing takes place.

It takes both courage and humility to seek mental health treatment. Regardless of what people know, the illness feels like personal failure, deep inadequacy, and a repulsive hidden blight. People generally do not seek treatment until every other effort has failed, every other avenue has been exhausted. Even in desperation, it takes great courage to approach a stranger with such great vulnerability, and to utter the obvious truth that I, too, need help. As clinicians, we need to remember and respect the daunting and powerful act that brings our patients to us for the first time, and begins the process of healing before we intervene. And we need to approach patients and the public in the same way: with humility and courage.

We are all familiar with the old 12-step adage "It's not your fault, but it's your responsibility." As professionals, we have an obligation to repeatedly reassure patients and families that no form of mental illness is their fault, regardless of their mistakes and failings. And we have an additional responsibility: to address the painful ways in which mental health professionals have added to the blame and shame of those with mental illness. I doubt that anyone reading this book contributed to the idea of the "schizophrenogenic mother" or regularly told patients things such as "You want to be depressed." But when we speak to laypersons, we represent all mental health professionals, past and present. It is our responsibility to address the well-intentioned but destructive mistakes of our past and even to apologize for them. It is our responsibility to show humility and a determination to set things right.

As we acknowledge and address old wounds, a deeper healing and a more powerful alliance forms. Nearly every time I speak publicly about mental illness, addressing this aspect of our past receives the biggest response. Audience members regularly approach me after the talk, explaining that they too felt blamed for mental illness in clinical settings. It is not important to know what the professionals actually said or meant to say. It is only important to acknowledge the deep effects of such wounds, and to address them with courtesy and respect. Mental illness is no one's fault, and this is a truth that liberates everyone: clinicians, family members, and those dealing with illness.

Mental Illness: Good News or Bad News?

Mental illness is common, so common that it affects us all (see Chapter 3). Mental illness is real, as real as any medical illness. It affects the brain, the immune system, the digestive system, the circulatory system, and the hormone system. It alters the body and effects almost every organ system in it (see Chapter 5). Mental illness kills people at a rate that rivals most other types of illness, and disables people more than most other types. It shortens the lifespan and makes people vulnerable to other illnesses such as diabetes and heart disease. Mental illness speeds up the aging process, taking a long-term toll on body and brain (see Chapter 6). Mental illness is serious business, by any medical or human standard. It represents a public health crisis of massive proportions, with a massive cost to society and a massive amount of human suffering.

Clearly, all of this represents bad news. It sums up, very inadequately, the burdens of countless millions of people dealing with mental illness right now. Countless people right now are disabled, exhausted, isolated, and in horrible pain due to mental illness. Countless people are in such a tormented, hopeless state that they are considering suicide. Countless people are getting little support and understanding to help them cope. Countless people have inadequate funding for their treatment and are living in poverty due to mental illness. And most of them have family members carrying an equal burden of pain and anxiety on behalf of those they love. Countless more have already lost family members to mental illness and live with the grief and guilt that this entails.

This is not good news, and it is overwhelming at times. But it is not the end of the story about mental illness—it is only the beginning. Facing the truth about mental illness is painful, but the truth is always liberating in the end. Just knowing the truth about mental illness helps people deal more successfully with it and eases the burdens on their families (Yesufu-Udechuku et al. 2015; Zhao et al. 2015). Facing the truth as a society is helping us transform the way we treat people with mental illness and address it more effectively than ever before in history. But facing the truth means facing the whole truth, not just the negative side of the truth. As human beings, we tend to pay more attention to the negative side of things than the positive side, but to get the whole truth, we need both sides (Ito et al. 1998). Therefore, for the rest of the book, I focus on the positive side of the truth about mental illness. And for many people, the positive side of the truth is just as difficult to believe as the negative side. Thus, we need to make sure we spend as much time thinking about the positive as the negative, for the sake of the truth and for the sake of our ability to keep going. Seeing the positive side gives us hope, a sense of progress, a sense that all this sacrifice will ultimately be worthwhile.

I know all of this from personal experience. I have suffered from mental illness, I have had family members suffer from mental illness, and I work with mental illness every day. I understand the pain of lives derailed, hopes destroyed, careers disrupted, and bodies devastated. I know the terror of uncontrollable illness and the permanent pain of losing people to mental health conditions. I know the relentless grind of chronic illness, of waiting months and years and even decades for things to improve, even a little bit. Yet I do not ultimately find my existence despairing. I do not find the lives of those with mental illness to be dispiriting. I find them to be inspiring. Every day I see victories, and every day I see hope. Every day I see people of extraordinary courage who simply will not give up, and every day I see many of them turning the tide on mental illness. I look around and see the science growing and society changing. I do not feel despair, and I believe that everyone who cares about mental illness must somehow share my hope and optimism. Otherwise, how could so many go on, waging this war on mental illness in the clinics, in public forums, and in private homes in every community?

The rest of this book represents the progress made by people with mental illness, family members, caring friends, mental health professionals, researchers, and advocates. All of them together have brought us to a better place, one that is unrecognizable compared to 100 years ago. Medically, socially, and scientifically, things are incomparably better, and we owe a debt of gratitude to those who brought us to this point. The best way we can repay their efforts is by recognizing and treasuring the progress they have brought us, then building on it going forward. And there is much to appreciate, much to celebrate, and much to take forward into the future.

Obviously, the most important good news about mental illness has to do with developments involving treatment. Ultimately, successful treatment is the best and only good news there is. Can we do something to ease the suffering of those with mental illness, to prevent the death and dysfunction that it brings? Can we someday cure or even prevent major mental illnesses? We will talk about treatment in Chapter 8, where we will see that the news is better than most people expect. But before we go there, we should spend some time on another bit of good news: Mental illness is nobody's fault.

This may seem quite weak for those needing good news. After all, the bad news is quite impressive. Mental illness is overwhelming in its ability to kill, disable, and decimate our health. How can it be equally good news that mental illness is nobody's fault? Who cares if someone is at fault when so many people have it? Who cares if someone is at fault when we just need to cure it? Why spend time arguing about who caused the problem when we just need to move on and fix it?

The Blame Game

The answer to these questions is an easy one for people with mental illness and their families: You too would care whose fault it was if you had been blamed for mental illness. For decades, people and families with mental illness suffered blame for the illnesses that tormented them. They will tell you why we have to talk about whose fault mental illness is: because the talking and fault-finding began many years ago. The conversation is an old one, and historically people with mental illness and their families have been the ones to receive the most blame for it.

The old saying about adding insult to injury does not remotely capture the pain that comes from being blamed for your own illness. Imagine being so desperate and tormented that you try to end your own life in a suicide attempt. Then imagine being in that state while emergency room staff treat you with coldness and contempt on top of all your other pain. Imagine the inner shame and chaos that someone feels who is overwhelmed by anxiety or hallucinations. Then imagine that after finally admitting you need help, you are told that you did this to yourself. Imagine being the parent of a child with devastating illness, and then being told you caused your child's incurable illness. People with mental illness and their families will tell you that the pain of this blame can be as bad as the pain of the illness, just as traumatizing and just as destructive. It is a big part of the shame and stigma that have hounded people with mental illness, and ending it will be a big part of lifting the stigma.

Blaming is not unique to mental illness. As human beings, we are prone to blame someone whenever something goes wrong. We pay more attention to negative events, and our brains react more strongly to negative than to positive events (Ito et al. 1998; Young et al. 2011). Even small children are more likely to blame others when something goes wrong than to credit them when something goes right (Leslie et al. 2006). Most people dislike negative political advertising, yet it persists. News media figured out a long time ago that people pay more attention to negative and anxiety-producing stories than positive ones (Soroka and McAdams 2015), which probably accounts for the approach to much of the news. So we should not be surprised that blame has continuously harried those who deal with mental illness. And plenty of people—families, medical professionals, and patients themselves—have been injured in the process.

Blaming Families

Not surprisingly, families have commonly been blamed for mental illness. Codependent families have been blamed for alcoholism and other addictions, and critical families have been blamed for depression and anxiety. But one family member—the mother—has been blamed more than any other, and one instance of this has done more harm than any other—the schizophrenogenic mother. *Schizophrenogenic* is a long and official-sounding term for something that begins schizophrenia. In the 1950s and 1960s, there was a theory that mothers who were especially difficult might trigger schizophrenia in their children (Fromm-Reichmann 1948). Such mothers were described as being controlling and cold and as placing their children in "double binds" through being simultaneously overprotective and rejecting. The schizophrenogenic mother theory persisted into the 1970s, and countless parents heard that they were to blame for their children's disabling and incurable illness. The pain and emotional trauma that they suffered from this stigma are difficult to imagine.

Happily, the theory faded into obscurity in the 1980s and has never resurfaced. It was always controversial, only one theory among many (Fry 1962; Higgins 1968), but it did a great deal of damage in its time. It was one example of a general assumption among mental health professionals that mental illnesses were learned patterns of behavior originating early childhood. According to the theory, preschool experiences created both personality and mental problems. Since parents were responsible for their children in early life, they had to be responsible for the mental and behavioral problems of their children. Even at the time, some mental health professionals warned against such assumptions (Chess 1964). One well-known psychiatrist published a famous paper coining the term "good-enough mother" (Winnicott 1953)—after all, what mother could be perfect? Other mental health experts maintained that mental illnesses were not learned at all, but purely biological (Gach 2008). Nevertheless, parents (and mothers in particular) were the "bad guys" of the mental health world for too many decades.

Mental health professionals, including psychiatrists, have been rightly criticized for this destructive assumption. Today, professionals cringe at the thought of blaming our greatest allies—the parents of people with mental illness (Harrington 2012). This should never have happened, and we psychiatrists owe a deep apology to all parents who suffered blame. Nevertheless, the theory did not reflect a failure of research. Instead, ongoing research eventually disproved the theory. Studies showed that the supposed "schizophrenogenic mother" was no more common among parents of people with schizophrenia than anyone else (Parker 1982).

Something else helped to put an end to the habit of blaming parents: Mental health advocacy by organizations such as Mental Health America and NAMI, the National Alliance on Mental Illness. NAMI was founded in 1979 by parents of adult children with schizophrenia, the very group that had previously been blamed for the problem. Parents, together with those who had mental illness, mounted a grassroots campaign to put an end to such blaming and educate the public about mental illness. They succeeded beyond their wildest dreams. They expected maybe 35 people at the first national NAMI conference, but 284 representatives from 59 organizations appeared, including prominent psychiatrists (National Institute on Mental Illness Wisconsin 2020). Today, NAMI has more than 168,000 members and is one of many important organizations transforming the way we deal with mental illness. So paradoxically, from one of the worst theories in mental health history came one of the most decisive advances in the history of mental health.

Blaming Doctors: The Toxic Psychiatrist

All of us recognize the need for someone to "take the fall" for tragic events, and we all can understand why psychiatrists have often been "fall guys" for mental illness. It is not hard to imagine that mental health professionals get together in committees, make up ideas about mental illness, diagnose people who do not really have it, then give them toxic or never-ending treatments (see Chapter 4). Educated people have argued (and continue to argue) that most mental health symptoms are perpetuated by medicines or drag on endlessly because of talk therapy, and that all of this supports a multimillion-dollar industry more than it helps troubled people. Although such accusations may seem extreme, there is a long list of books (with more every year) that have titles like these: *We've Had a Hundred Years of Psychotherapy— And the World's Getting Worse* (Hillman and Ventura 1993) and *Toxic Psychiatry: Why Therapy, Empathy, and Love Must Replace the Drugs, Electroshock, and Biochemical Theories of the "New Psychiatry"* (Breggin 2015).

I know a great many people in the field of mental health, and very few of them seem to be in it for the money or power. Yes, psychiatrists have a well-deserved reputation of being weird, but almost every mental health professional I know genuinely wants to help people. Anyone with an M.D. can go into a higher-status or higher-paying specialty than psychiatry, just as anyone capable of getting a Ph.D. can go into a higher-paying field than psychology. Most mental health professionals I talk to go into the field because they or family members have experienced the reality of mental illness, and they want to do something about it. Why would we find all of this fascinating if it did not relate to us personally? If we had no experience of anxiety, depression, or addiction, why on earth would we spend our lives understanding and treating it? If we did not already love people who have mental illness, why would we feel so compelled to work with it?

Although larger and more systematic studies are needed, research so far shows that mental health professionals have higher rates of mental illness, mental distress, and trauma than average. It is possible that three-quarters of professionals in mental health fields have a lifetime history of mental illness, with much higher rates of childhood trauma and neglect than people in other professions (Elliott and Guy 1993; Nachshoni et al. 2008; Pope and Feldman-Summers 1992). Temperamentally, people working in mental health care tend to be more emotionally sensitive and vulnerable to negative emotions (Deary et al. 1996). Developmentally, one common theme among mental health professionals is the childhood role of being a mediator and caretaker in troubled families, a role that they continue in adulthood (DiCaccavo 2002; Nikcevic et al. 2007). I am not trying to imply that mental health professionals are saints. Quite obviously, they are people who have plenty of their own problems. My point is that most people working in mental health professions do so for deeply personal reasons, not mainly for money or prestige. They generally do so because they personally know the pain of mental illness, either in themselves or in close family members.

Blaming the Patient: "You Want to Be Sick"

The blame that doctors have endured for working with mental illness does not compare to the pain and stigma endured by people who have mental illness. Although there have been many exceptions, people with severe mental illness have generally been mocked or shunned throughout recorded history. They have been rejected, friendless, poverty-stricken, and homeless. They have been called bums, crazy, weird, evil, demon-possessed, and subhuman. When not ignored, they have been tied up, chained up, put in cages, locked in basements, and imprisoned in jails. They have suffered verbal abuse, beatings, torture, and involuntary surgery. They have been treated like animals, executed, starved, or forgotten. Among the most vulnerable people in society, they have had few defenders in past generations and have too few now. Their mistreatment and ostracism continue to this day. The treatment of individuals with mental illness is one of the great, mostly unsung tragedies of human history (Powers 2017).

Today, people with mental illness receive better treatment than at any previous time in recorded history. Yet their situation is grim, especially for those with severe forms of mental illness. People with mental illness are more likely to experience poverty (Muntaner et al. 1998). They are three to four times more likely to be victims of violence and crime than people without mental illness (Teplin et al. 2005). And they are more likely to be jailed. As of 2005, there were three times more people with severe mental illness in jail than in psychiatric hospitals. The number of mental hospital beds in the United States had shrunk from one for every 300 persons in the 1950s to one for every 3,000 persons today (Torrey et al. 2010). Also, the percentage of people with mental illness who are imprisoned has swelled. Studies estimate that 15% of male prisoners and 30% of female prisoners suffer from *severe* mental illness, and about half of individuals in prisons have been diagnosed with mental illness while in prison (Al-Rousan et al. 2017). Many more suffer from "milder" forms that are still disabling and deadly, including posttraumatic stress disorder (PTSD) and addictions. While in prison, people with mental illness are more likely to suffer both sexual assault and physical assault than the average prisoner. The suicide rate among prisoners is reportedly three to six times higher than in the general population (Fazel et al. 2016).

Even for individuals with moderate and mild forms of mental illness, the road has not been easy. For a long time, therapists and doctors thought that patients might be at fault when they failed to improve with treatment. From the 1950s into the 1980s, most (though not all) educated people believed that mental illnesses were learned behaviors that people could change through self-improvement. There was a great deal of truth in this view, and it empowered many millions to address their own personal problems. The theory implied that people "learned" mental illness in childhood, so at least they were not to blame for having it in the first place. The underlying idea was that people with mental illness had it in their power to get better, and those who did not were often thought to be perpetuating their own illness. At some deep level, they were "choosing" to be sick rather than get well. In this sense, the theory blamed people for failing to cure themselves of mental illness.

One example of this belief involved the treatment of depression. People were told that they "wanted" to be depressed or disabled, that they were "self-sabotaging," and that they were trying to avoid responsibility or get attention. Best sellers on depression (even some that were generally good) had such titles as "Happiness Is a Choice" (Minirth and Meier 1978). Doctors regularly thought patients were looking for "secondary gain," referring to all the extra sympathy and help that came from being sick. Many doctors (including quite a few therapists) thought that depression was "anger turned inward" or even masochism, an underlying desire for pain and defeat (Burns 1981). The implication was that depressed people had to learn to stand up for themselves and express anger. In one mental hospital where I worked, there were old stories that depressed patients had once been sent to clean out bathrooms with a toothbrush and do other humiliating jobs, in hopes of "activating their anger." This, interestingly enough, was supposed to help them get out of depression.

Although those days are long past, people today still hear things like "Do you really want to get better?" (Borchard 2018), "Just exercise!" (McColl 2018), and "Stop feeling sorry for yourself" (Time to Change 2012). My personal favorite is "Stop being so negative" (McLaren 2017). Ah, how easy the job of a mental health professional would be if such comments cured mental illness! Of course, there is truth in the ideas that people can help depression with more exercise, more positive thinking, and less self-negativity. But when a depressed person hears such well-meaning advice, the unintended message is this: "You would not be depressed if only you did things right." And similar experiences have been described by those who have other kinds of mental illness. As the comedian Mitch Hedberg put it, "Alcoholism is the only disease where they yell at you for having it."

Ending the Blame Game: What Causes Mental Illness?

Today, we know what causes mental illness. Although we do not know all the details of how each mental illness is triggered, we do know the cause of mental illness in general. And it is very simple: **The cause of mental illness is genes plus stress.** Mental illness would not exist if people did not have genes to make them susceptible to mental illness. And regardless of anyone's genetics, mental illness would not develop if people did not have stress to trigger it.

We cannot blame people for their mental illness because no one picks their genes and no one picks their stresses. We don't choose our parents, and we aren't given a checklist of which genes we do and don't want. We all get the DNA we have as it randomly mixes through our parents. We don't choose to have a risk of schizophrenia, just as we don't choose to have a risk of heart attacks. Likewise, no one asks us what stressors we would like in life. No one asks when we would like our mother to die, when we should be in a car accident, or when we should have a bad day at work. Tomorrow morning when we wake up, we likely won't know what is going to happen to stress us during the day and whether it will be an easy or a hard day. We do not pick our stresses, any more than we pick our genes. We simply cope with them the best we can.

After all this talk about the brain's complexity, "genes plus stress" might sound too simple. Could that be the whole explanation? Let's first look at genes in more detail, then do the same for stress.

Genes

Although genes make mental illness possible, genes do not doom a person to mental illness. For example, having genes for an illness like schizophrenia does not mean that a person will get the illness. People with two parents who have schizophrenia get a lot of genes for schizophrenia, yet only about 50% of those offspring get the disease. The same is true for identical twins: If one has schizophrenia, there is a 50% chance that the other does as well (Riley and Kendler 2006). This percentage is high, but nowhere near 100%. Take the example of another illness, PTSD. A person cannot get PTSD without having had at least one traumatic experience. So the severe stress of trauma is an absolute necessity for the illness. Interestingly, the vast majority of people (about 70%) have experienced trauma (Kessler et al. 2017), but only a minority, about 7% of the population, get PTSD (Kessler and Wang 2008). Why? The reasons are complex, but they almost certainly include genetics (Smoller 2016). People with the right genes have a low risk of developing PTSD, even after a lot of trauma. Other people may be quite sensitive to adverse experiences and get PTSD with less intense traumas. Therefore, genes give us a risk of mental illness, but they alone do not give us mental illness. DNA is not destiny.

Why is this so? Because there is no single gene for any specific mental illness. Instead, there are hundreds of different genes that play into different mental illnesses, with most making a small contribution to the risk. Even with a heavy genetic risk of mental illness, some people never develop that mental illness. Genes alone are not enough. Experience (our interaction with the environment) plays a decisive part. Experience even turns genes on and off, causing them to be expressed or lie dormant in the DNA (Nestler et al. 2016). Experience plus genes determines the physical wiring and functioning of our brains as well. So stress and genes must literally interact for mental illness to develop.

Stress

How do we best understand stress? By remembering that it is both physically and mentally real. We all know what stress feels like mentally: We feel upset, tense, tired, negative, distracted, and so on. As we feel these things, our bodies are having a physical stress reaction. On the physical side, stress changes our hormones (especially cortisol), our brain transmitters (such as norepinephrine), our immunity, and our inflammation levels.

Stress is a normal part of life, shared by all people and mammals. In biological terms, stress is just an organism's response to change (Selye 1950). Whenever we have uncontrollable or unpredictable change, we have stress (Koolhaas et al. 2011). More change (good or bad) means more stress. Like change, stress is a necessary part of life. People usually handle stress pretty well, at least for short periods of time. Ongoing stress is another matter. Long-term or chronic stress has long-term effects on the body, as is evident in "before" and "after" photos of most U.S. presidents. Chronic stress puts us at risk for mental illness, as well as many other kinds of illness. It affects our brains, our hearts, our blood sugar, and every other organ system in the body. Long-term stress raises the risk of heart attacks, high blood pressure, infections, and diabetes, and it can worsen the course of illnesses such as cancer and arthritis (Dougall and Baum 2011).

Clearly, many different things can cause stress. For instance, psychological stress can occur when we are criticized and humiliated at work, or unhappy at home. Physical stress can occur in all sorts of ways, from lack of sleep to changes in diet to physical injury. Infection is a physical stress. So is exposure to hazardous chemicals such as lead and mercury. All types of stresses, not only psychological stress, play into mental illness. For instance, there is good evidence that infection in the developing brain may be an important risk factor for schizophrenia (Anderson and Maes 2013), but so are other stresses, such as nutritional problems, childhood trauma, and later use of marijuana (Davis et al. 2016). Physical stresses also affect depression and anxiety disorders. As discussed in Chapter 5, changes in gut bacteria may be important in increasing the risk of depression and anxiety. Many other physical illnesses, such as chronic pain and diabetes, are also risk factors. So are negative and stressful experiences, especially trauma and abuse (Li et al. 2016). Social situations like poverty and unemployment add to the chances of getting depression and other mental illnesses (Alegría et al. 2018). In other words, physical, mental, psychological, social, and environmental stressors can all be factors in mental illness, because all of them affect the whole person, body and mind.

Devil's Advocate: Why Shouldn't We Blame Those With Mental Illness?

Given enough of the wrong genes and the wrong stresses, anyone will develop mental illness. Mental illness is not a choice, as is true for any other kind of illness. We cannot control our own genes, and we cannot eliminate stress and trauma from life. So we cannot blame anyone for mental illness. Yet some people still have a nagging feeling that someone really is to blame for mental illness. Don't people do things that play into their own illnesses? After all, many people do things that make their own lives more stressful. People drink too much alcohol, smoke cigarettes, eat poorly, avoid exercise, overwork, and become sleep deprived. People think and act in negative and destructive ways. Don't these habits worsen our health? Don't these things play into mental illness?

We don't even need to limit the argument about blame to mental illnesses. Do people who smoke tobacco "deserve" in some way to get lung cancer or emphysema? Do people who eat poorly and gain weight "deserve" to get diabetes? People who are stressed out, sleeping poorly, and not exercising do seem to be putting themselves at higher risk for heart attacks. Who says they are *not* to blame?

This line of speculation makes sense, up to a point: Having a lot of stress raises the risk of depression and anxiety. Smoking marijuana raises the risk of schizophrenia. People cannot become addicted to alcohol if they never drink alcohol. So maybe bad habits lead to mental illnesses, just as bad habits lead to a lot of physical illnesses. Why aren't people with illnesses to blame for all of this?

The reason we cannot blame people for their illnesses is the following: *Stress is normal, but illness is not a normal consequence of stress. Illness is an abnormal breakdown in the body's functioning in response to stress.* In other words, stress is always part of life. Everyone has stress. There is no stress-free living. Likewise, everyone has bad habits: Some people drink too much alcohol, but some people work too hard. Some people do not get up and exercise, and some people never take time to relax. Some people worry too much, whereas other people do not plan ahead. But no one is perfect, and everyone has bad habits. So people who develop illnesses, including mental illnesses, are no different from everyone else. Everyone has stress, but for some people stress leads to anxiety or depression. For others, it leads to heart attacks or high blood pressure. There is nothing that makes those people worse than anyone else. Almost everyone tries alcohol at some point in life, but most people do not become addicted. Those people who did not get addicted to alcohol are not "better" than someone who did. Some people do not get enough sleep and have strokes, whereas other people do not get enough sleep and become manic. Stress and bad habits are common to us all. Depending on our genetics and development, some of us will get illnesses sooner, and some of us will get illnesses later. But all of us will eventually get illnesses, and all of us will have some bad habits that play into stress and illness. Whether these bad habits and stresses play into mental or physical illnesses is a matter of genetics plus the developmental course of our lives. None of us can point the finger at people who have mental illness and say that they deserve it more than the rest of us.

If people who *get* mental illness aren't to blame, what about people who *give* mental illness to others? Parents abuse their children and "give" them PTSD. People who commit crimes like rape and assault can also cause others to get PTSD. And abusive people put others at risk for many mental illnesses, not only PTSD. Abuse and other traumas contribute to depression, anxiety, addiction, and even schizophrenia. So can we say that abusive people are to blame for the mental illness they cause? Yes and no. Yes, abusive people have done terrible wrongs, and they are morally responsible for the wrongs they cause. A drunk driver who runs over someone is in the wrong and responsible for that crime and for the medical problems of the victim, including PTSD. But what about a drunk driver who narrowly missed running over someone? Is the second drunk driver better than the first? No, the two drivers are equally wrong and equally bad in that moment. They are equally to blame. The fact that someone experienced a consequence such as broken bones or PTSD in one case but not the other does not add to or subtract from the wrong that was done, even though it adds to the damage. The person who caused the illness has greater *responsibility* but no more *blame* than the person who did not. Both have blame, but one has more responsibility. In the same way, all parents who are abusive should have equal *blame*, and all have responsibility for the consequences of the abuse. But parents who cause mental illness have an additional *responsibility* to help heal that illness.

Blame Versus Responsibility

What about people who have mental illness? Are they responsible? Yes, but in a completely different way. As Alcoholics Anonymous has said for decades, it is not our fault if we have an illness, but it is our responsibility to do something about it. All of us have responsibility for our own health. None of us handles our health perfectly, but all of us have a responsibility to seek health care when we are sick, to accept the treatment we need, and to learn about how to take care of ourselves. All of us are responsible for making our own health care decisions, and all of us are responsible for the consequences of our decisions. It is up to us to face our problems and illnesses, and to do something about them.

During severe mental illness, people may lose the ability to exercise this sacred responsibility for themselves. Some can become so paranoid that they cannot trust anyone, including doctors and families. Others can become so manic that they literally cannot see the problems that are destroying their lives. Severe mental illness can disable our ability to focus and reason, and shut down our ability to make our usual kinds of decisions. Some people's mental illness even keeps them from recognizing their own mental illness.

This is a difficult problem, but it is still comparable to what occurs with other medical illnesses. There are many medical illnesses that make people confused, unconscious, or unable to make decisions in their usual way. For instance, when someone arrives at the emergency department unconscious and injured from a car accident, physicians assume that person wants treatment and do not delay giving it. Likewise, when someone is in a coma or has a head injury, physicians assume the person wants treatment unless close family says otherwise. Once the patient is back to a normal state, the patient can accept or refuse treatment. The same thing applies to mental illness. When people are unable to understand the basic realities of their illness and treatment, then mental health professionals assume the people want treatment. Once they are better and in a condition to make their own decisions, however, they have the right to make their treatment decisions for themselves.

Obviously, our society has not yet worked out how to apply these principles in every case. Many family members live with a person who has severe mental illness but refuses treatment because of the mental illness. These situations are gut-wrenching and heartbreaking and involve terrible choices for family members. But none of this changes the fact that mental illness is another form of medical illness and should be treated the same way. None of it changes the fact that no one is to blame for mental illness. Parents and families are not to blame. Doctors are not to blame. People with mental illness are not to blame. Society is not to blame. All of us, in our own way, are responsible. But the tragedy of mental illness is no one's fault. It is part of the tragedy of life. It is a part of the human condition, a condition that all of us share. So we should treat everyone accordingly, especially those who have the misfortune of mental illness.

Advice for Advocacy

- A little apology goes a long way with people who are suspicious of mental health care.

- Apologizing for mistakes of the past does not mean painting previous mental health care with a broad brush. Many generations of professionals have worked and sacrificed to help those with mental illness. They used the best tools available to them at the time.

- Thus, be wary of narratives that divide people into good and bad groups during the history of mental health care. Patients, families, and professionals have all been wrongly blamed for mental illness and have all contributed to better treatment of those with illness. We are all in the same boat.

- When using "genes plus stress" as a shorthand for the cause of mental illness, remember that stress is not limited to psychological events here. It includes social, environmental, and medical (biological) stressors as well.

- It is important to stress that genes do not equal destiny. Many of the lay public and even academics assume that genetic contributions to mental illness imply genetic determinism—fixed outcomes regardless of environment. This misunderstanding must often be explicitly addressed.

- No one is to blame for mental illness," is a bold statement. Some mental health professionals will want to make exceptions for abusive or irresponsible people who traumatize others. Whether they do so will depend on their definition of "blame" in this context.

References

Alegría M, NeMoyer A, Bagué IF, et al: Social determinants of mental health: where we are and where we need to go. Cur Psychiatry Rep 20(11):95, 2018

Al-Rousan T, Rubenstein L, Sieleni B, et al: Inside the nation's largest mental health institution: a prevalence study in a state prison system. BMC Public Health 17(1):342, 2017

Anderson G, Maes M: Schizophrenia: linking prenatal infection to cytokines, the tryptophan catabolite (TRYCAT) pathway, NMDA receptor hypofunction, neurodevelopment and neuroprogression. Prog Neuropsychopharmacol Biol Psychiatry 42:5–19, 2013

Borchard T: Do you want to be depressed? PsychCentral, July 8, 2018. Available at: https://psychcentral.com/blog/do-you-want-to-be-depressed. Accessed July 30, 2020.

Breggin P: Toxic Psychiatry: Why Therapy, Empathy and Love Must Replace the Drugs, Electroshock, and Biochemical Theories of the "New Psychiatry." New York, St. Martin's Press, 2015

Burns DD: Feeling Good. New York, Signet Books, 1981

Chess S: Mal de mère. Am J Orthopsychiatry 34(4):613–614, 1964

Davis J, Eyre H, Jacka FN, et al: A review of vulnerability and risks for schizophrenia: beyond the two hit hypothesis. Neurosci Biobehav Rev 65:185–194, 2016

Deary IJ, Agius RM, Sadler A: Personality and stress in consultant psychiatrists. Int J Soc Psychiatry 42(2):112–123, 1996

DiCaccavo A: Investigating individuals' motivations to become counselling psychologists: the influence of early caretaking roles within the family. Psychol Psychother 75(4):463–472, 2002

Dougall AL, Baum A: Stress, health, and illness, in Handbook of Health Psychology. Edited by Baum A, Revenson TA, Singer J. Abingdon, UK, Routledge, 2011, pp 321–337

Elliott DM, Guy JD: Mental health professionals versus non-mental-health professionals: childhood trauma and adult functioning. Professional Psychology: Research and Practice 24(1):83–90, 1993

Fazel S, Hayes AJ, Bartellas K, et al: Mental health of prisoners: prevalence, adverse outcomes, and interventions. Lancet Psychiatry 3(9):871–881, 2016

Fromm-Reichmann F: Notes on the development of treatment of schizophrenics by psychoanalytic psychotherapy. Psychiatry 11(3):263–273, 1948

Fry WF Jr: The schizophrenogenic "who." Psychoanalytic Review 49(4):68–73, 1962

Gach J: Biological psychiatry in the nineteenth and twentieth centuries, in History of Psychiatry and Medical Psychology. Edited by Wallace ER, Gach J. Boston, MA, Springer, 2008, pp 381–418

Harrington A: The fall of the schizophrenogenic mother. Lancet 379(9823):1292–1293, 2012

Higgins J: The schizophrenogenic mother revisited. British Journal of Psychiatric Social Work 9(4):205–208, 1968

Hillman J, Ventura M: We've Had a Hundred Years of Psychotherapy—and the World's Getting Worse. New York, HarperOne, 1993

Ito TA, Larsen JT, Smith NK, et al: Negative information weighs more heavily on the brain: the negativity bias in evaluative categorizations. J Pers Soc Psychol 75(4):887–900, 1998

Kessler RC, Wang PS: The descriptive epidemiology of commonly occurring mental disorders in the United States. Annu Rev Public Health 29:115–129, 2008

Kessler RC, Aguilar-Gaxiola S, Alonso J, et al: Trauma and PTSD in the WHO World Mental Health surveys. Eur J Psychotraumatol 8 (suppl 5):1353383, 2017

Koolhaas JM, Bartolomucci A, Buwalda B, et al: Stress revisited: a critical evaluation of the stress concept. Neurosci Biobehav Rev 35(5):1291–1301, 2011

Leslie AM, Knobe J, Cohen A: Acting intentionally and the side-effect effect: theory of mind and moral judgment. Psychol Sci 17(5):421–427, 2006

Li M, D'arcy C, Meng X: Maltreatment in childhood substantially increases the risk of adult depression and anxiety in prospective cohort studies: systematic review, meta-analysis, and proportional attributable fractions. Psychol Med 46(4):717–730, 2016

Mannarini S, Rossi A: Assessing mental illness stigma: a complex issue. Front Psychol 9:2722, 2019

McColl B: I have depression and anxiety. Please stop telling me to "go for a run." Self, April 16, 2018. Available at: www.self.com/story/depression-anxiety-exercise. Accessed July 30, 2020.

McLaren K: What I hear when you tell me to "stop being so negative." The Mighty, May 11, 2017. Available at: https://themighty.com/2017/05/stop-being-so-negative-depression. Accessed July 30, 2020.

Minirth FB, Meier PD: Happiness Is a Choice. Grand Rapids, MI, Baker Book House, 1978

Muntaner C, Eaton WW, Diala C, et al: Social class, assets, organizational control and the prevalence of common groups of psychiatric disorders. Soc Sci Med 47(12):2043–2053, 1998

Nachshoni T, Abramovitch Y, Lerner V, et al: Psychologists' and social workers' self-descriptions using DSM-IV psychopathology. Psychol Rep 103(1):173–188, 2008

National Institute on Mental Illness Wisconsin: History. 2020. Available at: https://namiwisconsin.org/about-nami-wisconsin/history. Accessed July 30, 2020.

Nestler EJ, Peña CJ, Kundakovic M, et al: Epigenetic basis of mental illness. Neuroscientist 22(5):447–463, 2016

Nikcevic AV, Kramolisova-Advani J, Spada MM: Early childhood experiences and current emotional distress: what do they tell us about aspiring psychologists? J Psychol 141(1):25–34, 2007

Parker G: Re-searching the schizophrenogenic mother. J Nerv Ment Dis 170(8):452–462, 1982

Pope KS, Feldman-Summers S: National survey of psychologists' sexual and physical abuse history and their evaluation of training and competence in these areas. Professional Psychology: Research and Practice 23(5):353–361, 1992

Powers R: No One Cares About Crazy People: The Chaos and Heartbreak of Mental Health in America. New York, Hachette Books, 2017

Riley B, Kendler KS: Molecular genetic studies of schizophrenia. Eur J Hum Genet 14(6):669–680, 2006

Selye H: Stress and the general adaptation syndrome. Br Med J 1(4667):1383–1392, 1950

Smoller JW: The genetics of stress-related disorders: PTSD, depression, and anxiety disorders. Neuropsychopharmacology 41(1):297–319, 2016

Soroka S, McAdams S: News, politics, and negativity. Political Communication 32(1):1–22, 2015

Teplin LA, McClelland GM, Abram KM, et al: Crime victimization in adults with severe mental illness: comparison with the National Crime Victimization Survey. Arch Gen Psychiatry 62(8):911–921, 2005

Time to Change: The same old comments: "stop feeling sorry for yourself." June 20, 2012. Available at: www.time-to-change.org.uk/blog/depression-same-old-comments. Accessed July 30, 2020.

Torrey EF, Kennard AD, Eslinger D, et al: More Mentally Ill Persons Are in Jails and Prisons Than Hospitals: A Survey of the States. Arlington, VA, Treatment Advocacy Center, 2010

Winnicott DW: Transitional objects and transitional phenomena—a study of the first not-me possession. Int J Psychoanal 34(2):89–97, 1953

Yesufu-Udechuku A, Harrison B, Mayo-Wilson E, et al: Interventions to improve the experience of caring for people with severe mental illness: systematic review and meta-analysis. Br J Psychiatry 206(4):268–274, 2015

Young L, Scholz J, Saxe R: Neural evidence for "intuitive prosecution": the use of mental state information for negative moral verdicts. Soc Neurosci 6(3):302–315, 2011

Zhao S, Sampson S, Xia J, et al: Psychoeducation (brief) for people with serious mental illness. Cochrane Database Syst Rev (4):CD010823, 2015

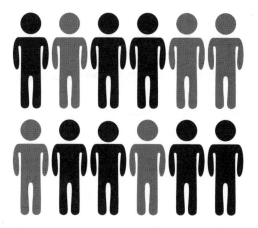

8

Mental Illness Is Treatable

Half Truth: We do not have cures for mental illness.

Whole Truth: Although we do not have cures, our treatments for mental illness are generally as good as our treatments for other chronic illnesses such as high blood pressure and diabetes.

Important Points

- In general, mental illnesses are chronic illnesses, like diabetes or migraine headaches. Chronic illnesses are long lasting but do not usually kill us quickly.
- In general, we do not have cures for chronic illnesses, and we do not have cures for mental illness.
- Although we have no cures, we do have effective treatments for mental illnesses, as we do for other common medical illnesses.

- Statistically speaking, medications for mental illnesses are just as likely to be helpful as medicines for other chronic diseases.
- In addition to effective medications, we have many other scientifically proven treatments, such as talk therapy and group treatments. Some are as effective as medications.
- Mental health treatments are complementary: They can work better when combined than they do individually.

Introduction

Psychiatry's aura of inferiority stems from many sources, but two in particular dog mental health professionals: First, we do not fully understand the disorders we treat. Second, we cannot cure the disorders we treat. These two notions have implicitly branded those who work with mental illness as second-class professionals, people who have commendable compassion but lack the true expertise and technical power of modern-day doctors and health care providers. In short, we bring good will but not efficacy to our patients.

In my opinion, this impression of our work is more damaging to patients than any other kind of stigma. It creates an imaginary dark cloud of despair over all mental health treatment. Given the level of pessimism about treatment that I see in patients who do show up for care, I can only imagine the hopelessness of those who do not. Most people do not seek mental health treatment, and most of those who do give up on treatment prematurely. In my attendance at a variety of advocacy events, I see no evidence of an overabundance of optimism.

However, the belief that mental health treatment is hopeless or even inferior is demonstrably false. It provides yet another example of how critics evaluate psychiatry by a different standard than other branches of medicine. Critics and even advocates often forget that mental health professionals treat *chronic* illnesses, and then they compare our treatments with those for *acute* illnesses. Granted, mental health treatments do not provide the routine rapid responses of antibiotics or surgeries. But neither do treatments for other chronic medical illnesses that are directly comparable to mental illness. Treatments for diabetes, heart disease, and a host of other chronic illnesses hardly amount to cures, and the most effective combinations of treatment often involve "lifestyle changes" such as exercise and stress management. Social factors are also profoundly important for successful treatment of these illnesses. When evaluated as treatment of chronic illness, mental health treatment fares quite well compared with other branches of medicine.

In short, psychiatric treatment is scientifically real and is comparable to treatments of other common chronic illnesses. This insight alone will do more to energize patients, families, advocates, and decision makers than any other. If we professionals can dispel the widespread and false belief that our treatments are more damaging than effective, we can permanently alter the landscape of mental health treatment.

What Doctors Don't Know

Finally, we have arrived at the most important chapter in this book. If you have any interest in mental health, then you already knew that mental illness is important. You already knew it is common. You already knew that it is real. You probably already knew that it is a medical illness, that it is physical as well as psychological. But many people who care about mental illness have not been told just how treatable it is. In fact, many medical doctors have not heard the best news about mental illness. I come from a family of medical doctors, and talk to other kinds of doctors on a regular basis. None of them ever express doubt about the reality of mental illness. Every medical doctor goes through a psychiatry rotation during medical school, and each one whom I know recognizes mental illness as another form of medical illness. This in itself is great news. Doctors and other medical professionals do not doubt the reality of mental illness. On the other hand, many doctors from other specialties lack a sense of how much we can do for mental illness. Many seem to feel sorry for me as a psychiatrist. "I could never go into psychiatry," they say with a frown. "I could not stand seeing people month after month, year after year, without any improvement. Patients coming back for the same thing over and over, with the same symptoms and the same complaints—I have to feel like I am curing people. I want to make a difference. That's why I went into medicine!"

I usually just smile in response to these kinds of comments. I am happy enough that most medical doctors now treat psychiatrists as fellow doctors, instead of "witch doctors" and "head shrinks." I am happy that my fellow physicians see people with mental illness as people who have medical conditions. And I am happy that other medical specialists treat more cases of mental illness than psychiatrists themselves. But even many of the doctors prescribing medication and psychotherapy for mental illness do not realize the power of the treatments they prescribe. If they did, they too would smile when they think about treating mental illness.

What Doctors Want

When I was a young psychiatrist seeing patients in the psychiatric hospital, one of my psychiatrist colleagues (Dr. Ty Porter) had a running joke. Every time I asked him how he was doing, he would reply, "I'm doing great. Saving lives and stamping out mental illness!" This always made me smile, but our work did not feel so triumphant at the time. We worked in a crisis psychiatric unit, and every day we would admit people who were psychotic and agitated, on the brink of suicide, or completely unable to function. We had only a few days to try and "patch them up," to help stabilize them, and to set them up for longer-term treatment. Like most psychiatric hospital units today, it was a short-term mental health unit. It did not feel like we were stamping out mental illness. It felt like we were hanging on for dear life and hoping our patients would as well.

Indeed, this type of work was a long way from the medicine that most doctors dream of practicing. Most medical doctors really do want to save lives and stamp out illness. That is the way things seem to work in movies and television shows, anyway: People come into the hospital in desperate straits, and the doctor knows just what to do to cure them. The doctor leans over the patient, shines a light in the eyes, and then starts barking out decisive orders for lab tests and treatments. The doctor stops the bleeding, sews up the wound, does an operation, transfuses blood, or gives a life-saving antibiotic. Real medical doctors seem to like this image every bit as much as the general public. Doctors want to see themselves as people who cure illnesses, and like the idea of curing patients quickly and decisively.

There is nothing wrong with this image. When we are sick, we like the idea of doctors (and other health professionals) jumping in to cure us. When we are frightened and ill, we want to know that we will get better. And curing illnesses is exactly what medical professionals are supposed to do. But curing illness is only a part of medicine, and it turns out that dramatic cures are only a small part of the picture. Today, extraordinary medical treatments are available, and doctors can cure many kinds of illness. However, most doctors cannot cure most of the people they see. This is not because they are bad doctors using bad medicines—the difficulty lies in the nature of the illnesses themselves.

The Reality of Medicine: Acute Versus Chronic Illness

Medicine today cannot cure the majority of cases of illness that are seen in clinics. Doctors cannot cure the majority of important public health problems today. As a doctor, I would like to think we could. But in fact, we can only regularly cure one kind of illness: acute illness. Acute illness comes on quickly and goes away quickly. The flu is an acute illness. If you have the flu today, you are not going to have it 3 months from now. If you have a healthy immune system, your body's defenses will kick in and you will get over the flu within a few weeks. The same is true of another acute illness, a broken leg. If your leg is broken today, it is not likely to be broken a year from now. It may heal poorly or heal well, but it will heal. A cut or other injury will heal too. A heart attack is a life-threatening emergency, but it will not go on for very long. All of these are short-term or acute illnesses.

Technically speaking, an acute illness will get better or kill you within a limited amount of time. Sadly, the flu kills people every year, although most of us get over the flu without complications. If you are injured in a car accident, you are likely to recover, although of course you might not survive. There is a saying in emergency rooms that I do not like to repeat, because it is a dark kind of humor appreciated only by overworked doctors and nurses, but it nevertheless reflects the truth about acute illness: "All bleeding stops—eventually." In other words, our natural defenses will start clotting to stop the bleeding, but if they fail—and if medical treatment fails— a person can bleed to death. This is the uncomfortable and dramatic nature of acute illnesses. They either go away or kill you.

Most doctors I know love to treat acute illnesses. It is very satisfying to sew up a cut or knock out an infection with an antibiotic. Surgeons love to operate, because they can go in and fix the problem, right then and there. Cardiologists can often dissolve clots or open clogged arteries, stopping a heart attack on the spot. This makes everyone feel good, both doctors and patients. But the important point about acute illness is that it will go away anyway. Acute illnesses do not last. They just heal better with treatment than without it.

Chronic illnesses, in contrast, tend to go on indefinitely. They do not kill us, or at least not rapidly. They do take a toll on our health and lifespan, and may eventually kill us. High blood pressure is a chronic illness, and so is coronary artery disease, the chronic illness behind heart attacks. Diabetes is another common example, and so is arthritis. Asthma, high cholesterol, and migraine headaches are chronic. Chronic illnesses are not any less serious and deadly than acute illnesses. They just last longer, going on for months and years instead of days and weeks.

The vast majority of medical spending, 90%, goes toward the treatment of chronic illnesses (Buttorff et al. 2017). Most doctors spend the majority of their time treating people with chronic illnesses. Of course, people with chronic illnesses have acute medical problems too, but more visits to doctors every year are for chronic medical problems than acute ones (Centers for Disease Control and Prevention 2016). In the United States, 60% of people have at least one chronic illness, and 42% have two or more chronic illnesses (Buttorff et al. 2017). Therefore, chronic illness is the norm, not the exception, both for the general population and for doctors (Figures 8–1 and 8–2).

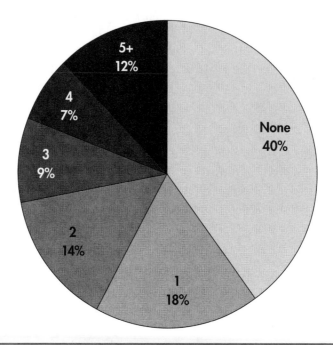

FIGURE 8–1. Percentage of Americans with 0–5+ chronic medical conditions.

60% of the population has at least one chronic illness; 42% has two or more.
Source.   Data from Buttorff et al. 2017.

All of us who live long enough will experience chronic illness for a significant portion of our lives. This may sound strange. Many older people seem healthy. I remember going to funerals as a kid where people would say, "He was never sick a day in his life." Oh, yes, he was. He may not have had symptoms, but he had a chronic illness whether anyone knew it or not. He may have had heart disease long before his heart attack, or maybe high blood pressure and high cholesterol long before his stroke. But for those of us who live long enough, chronic illness is just part of life.

The medical treatments we have today are better at treating acute illness than chronic illness. We are better at treating the flu and appendicitis than we are at treating high blood pressure and diabetes. We have cures for a good many acute illnesses, but not for many chronic illnesses. Unfortunately, most of the illnesses that are hurting most people today are chronic. Two-thirds of the world's deaths are now due to chronic illnesses, and chronic illness is the primary cause of poor health, disability, and death in the United States (Bauer et al. 2014). Our top health problems—heart disease, diabe-

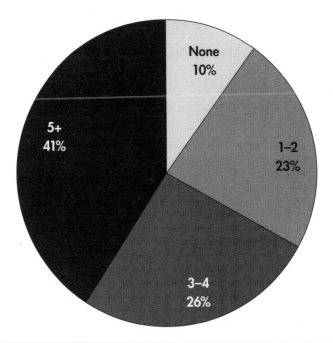

FIGURE 8–2. Percentage of medical spending by number of chronic medical conditions.

Source.   Data from Buttorff et al. 2017.

tes, and cancer—are all chronic health problems. So are other important public health problems such as arthritis, emphysema, asthma, high blood pressure, and obesity. Yet with the exception of some kinds of cancer, we do not have cures for any of these. We cannot cure diabetes or heart disease or even high blood pressure. Despite the lack of cures, no one should despair. We have good treatments for most chronic illnesses, and everyone who has one of these conditions should see the doctor for possible treatment.

The same applies to mental illnesses. Most cases of mental illness turn out to be chronic and relapsing. Except in the case of suicide, mental illness does not kill people quickly. But it disables people, takes a toll on health, and leads to earlier death. Mental illness is a unique type of chronic illness, but it shares many of the characteristics of other chronic illnesses. The most important is that it is not curable. We can't cure most mental illnesses (although there are exceptions), but we can most definitely treat them. On the other hand, most of us know of cases of mental illness that did not respond well to treatment. So let's look at just how treatable mental illness is compared to other chronic illnesses.

Treatment Efficacy: Mental Illnesses Versus Other Medical Illnesses

Although some people might think of most medical illnesses as curable and of mental illnesses as untreatable, this is not the case. Instead, mental illness and most kinds of chronic illness are treatable, but few are curable. Good treatments are available for diabetes and heart disease, as well as for depression and addiction. But most people would say that the treatments for mental illness are weak, even questionable, and some people write books claiming that mental health treatment is a fraud (see Chapter 4). So how does mental health treatment stack up against other medical treatments?

Happily, science has a way to examine this question. The answer lies in a common medical measurement called *efficacy*. Efficacy is simply a number that indicates the effectiveness of a given treatment. How much does this treatment do what we hope it will do? Efficacy measures the answer to this question. The scale of efficacy (technically the "Hedges' g") is around 0 to 1. I say "around" 0 to 1 because efficacy can be lower than 0 or higher than 1. A number anywhere near 0, such as 0.1 or 0.2, represents a weak treatment. The treatment may do as much harm as good, or do little to help the problem. On the other hand, efficacy near 1, say 0.7 or 0.8, represents a very effective treatment, something close to a home run for that medical condition. In the middle, around 0.4 to 0.6, are moderately effective treatments. These are good, strong, solid medical treatments, but they are not near cures.

All this is quite abstract, but if you understand this particular bit of research, you are likely to find the results as stunning and encouraging as I do. So here it is: One team of researchers decided to compare the efficacy of mental health medications against the efficacy of other common medical treatments (Leucht et al. 2012). The idea was to compare common medicines used in primary care to common medicines used in mental health care. For instance, if you go see your primary doctor for a common medical condition, like migraine headaches or high cholesterol, you might well walk out with a prescription for a medication. On the other hand, if you see a psychiatrist for a mental health condition like anxiety or schizophrenia, you might also walk out with a prescription. So which prescription is likely to be more effective? On average, will a prescription for a mental illness be more powerful, or a prescription for some common general medical condition?

In order to answer this question, the researchers assembled 94 different meta-analyses involving hundreds of studies with many thousands of patients. They compared efficacy for 48 drugs treating 20 common *medical* conditions,

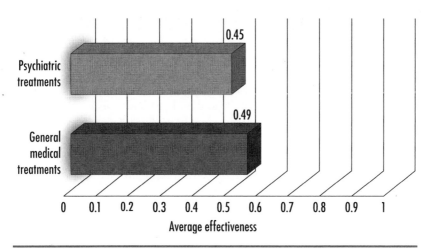

FIGURE 8–3. Comparing average effectiveness of general medical and mental health medications.

Source. Data from Leucht et al. 2012.

things like high blood pressure, migraine headaches, and breast cancer. They came up with an average efficacy for all these medication treatments, and then did the same analysis on the mental health side: They took 16 well-studied medicines for 8 different *mental* illnesses, and found an average efficacy for these treatments.

On average, are general medical treatments more effective than psychiatric treatments? Most people would guess that mental health medications do not work as well as others, but most people would be wrong. Medicines for mental health conditions have an average effectiveness of 0.45, while medicines for other common medical conditions average 0.49 (Leucht et al. 2012)—both are within the study's margin of error, so there is no statistically significant difference between the two (Figure 8–3). What does this mean? It means that *when you visit a psychiatrist (or other mental health provider) and walk out with a prescription, that prescription, on average, will be just as effective as a prescription from your primary care doctor for some other medical condition.* On average, a medicine for things like schizophrenia or social anxiety disorder will be as effective as a medicine for things like high blood pressure or migraine headaches.

On average, medications prescribed by a primary care doctor or by a mental health provider will not be cures, but they will be good, strong, solid treatments of moderate effectiveness. One is likely to be as effective as the other. So no one should brush off seeking mental health treatment by saying, "What's the point of going in for help? They'll just throw drugs or psychobabble at me and it won't do any good." Everyone with a significant mental illness should get treatment, just as everyone with a significant medical illness (of whatever kind) should get treatment. There is no reason to despair or give up.

At the same time, some of us can think of people who have not responded to treatment. What about people who died by suicide, or people who became psychotic and ran away? What about people who do not seem to improve with medicines? As a psychiatrist, I know the pain of working with people, trying treatment after treatment, and seeing no result. So regardless of the research, how can mental health treatments be effective medical treatments when many people do not respond? The answer is that mental health treatments are not exceptional among medical treatments. Like most medical treatments, they are effective most of the time but not all of the time. Even with good treatments available, people die of common medical illnesses. People die of high blood pressure, diabetes, and heart disease, even though we have good treatments for all of them. In the same way, people die of major depression, bipolar disorder, and addiction, even though we have good treatments for all of them.

This is a sad state of affairs for those who deal personally with mental illness, but it is important and comforting information for one group of people: people who have lost someone to mental illness. Most people who have seen a family member decline into permanent disability or die by suicide carry a tremendous burden of guilt. Suicide survivors in particular may bear an extra level of shame and torment over failing to prevent the suicide. Most will think repeatedly of their own "mistakes," things they desperately wish they had done differently. But mistakes are not the problem—mistakes are a normal and inevitable part of life. The problem is that sometimes people die of illnesses, even when the family does everything right, and even when the doctors and nurses do everything right. People die of mental illness even when they get good treatment, just like some people die of treatment-resistant high blood pressure or diabetes.

Mental Health Treatment: Much More Than Medicines

In spite of the challenges involved, the news about treatment is good. In fact, the news is even better than I previously described. We have been discussing mental health medications, which turn out to be as effective as other kinds of medicine. This is critically good news. But mental health treatment offers more than just medicine, which is even better news. Yes, medicines are typically required to treat moderate and severe mental illness, and they are an option with milder forms, namely for those who would rather take a medicine than do other kinds of treatment like psychotherapy. But no one is limited to medicine alone. Many other kinds of treatment for mental illness have been scientifically proven to work. Best of all, combining different forms of mental health treatment can lead to even better results. In many cases, medicine works better with psychotherapy (Huhn et al. 2014; Kamenov et al. 2017; Skapinakis et al. 2016), and exercise can give added benefit to medications (Firth et al. 2015) and possibly to talk therapy (Abdollahi et al. 2017). All of these treatments will probably work better when we provide people with additional social support and connection. This is great news about treatment of mental health conditions: We have many proven treatments, and we can use many of them at the same time. No one need despair.

Biological Versus Psychological Causes

Virtually all mental health professionals agree with what I have just said about treatment. But there was a time when mental health was divided into different warring camps, people who fundamentally disagreed about what good treatment meant. On one side were people who thought of mental illness and its treatment as completely *biological*. They thought that mental illnesses were biological, physical disorders of brain function, and that mental illnesses should only be treated biologically, using treatments such as medications and electroconvulsive therapy (ECT). They thought that psychotherapy (talk therapy) was unscientific, made-up psychobabble that was a waste of time and money. On the other side were people who thought that mental illnesses were completely *psychological*. They thought that medicines were toxic at worst and numbing at best and that medications just got in the way of good psychological treatment such as psychotherapy or support groups. They advised people to steer clear of biological psychiatry (Harrington 2019; Luhrmann 2001).

There were other camps as well, mostly outside of the mental health establishment. Some thought that mental illness was not any kind of illness, just an expression of *social* problems (such as poverty) or society's intolerance of nonconformists. They believed that social change and acceptance would take care of mental health conditions (Laing 1965; Scheff 1966). Finally, there were some religious people who thought that mental illnesses were not medical or mental problems, but instead were spiritual problems that could only be healed by spiritual growth or conversion (Koenig 2000; Stanford 2012).

Broadly speaking, the days of mental health factions are over. People dealing with mental illness now understand that all of us need all of the help we can get. Mental health professionals understand this, and those suffering from mental illness understand it. Some people are more interested in understanding or utilizing the biological approach, and some favor the psychological approach. But all points of view are relevant, and all approaches can be part of good mental health treatment. They are not in conflict with each other. Used correctly, all of them have the same goal: that of helping individuals with mental illness.

In the end, it turned out that all of the various groups were right, and all of them were wrong. Mental illness (as we have seen) is most definitely physical illness. And it is most definitely psychological illness that can be treated with psychological treatments. At the same time, social factors (such as poverty and inequality) are powerful factors in mental health, and the same can be said of spiritual factors. All of these—biological, psychological, social, and spiritual—have roles in mental illness, and all can be part of addressing mental illness. So in the rest of this chapter, we will look at each of these types of treatment.

Biological Treatments

The most common biological treatment for mental illness is medication. Proven medications are available for almost all major mental disorders. (One exception is phobias, such as fear of spiders, which respond well to behavioral psychotherapy.) When I say "proven," I mean proven in the way that any medical treatment should be proven. All medicines for mental health conditions go through the same rigorous process of testing as do medications for other medical conditions. They are evaluated in just the same way that the U.S. Food and Drug Administration (FDA) evaluates medicines for blood pressure or headache. No medications are approved without proof that they are reasonably safe and reasonably effective. And there are quite a few FDA-approved medicines for mental illness (Table 8–1).

For instance, there have been at least 522 well-performed studies (with a total of 116,477 people) showing that *antidepressants* have efficacy for depression (Cipriani et al. 2018). At least seven well-done studies (with 1,580 participants) have shown that *lithium* helps prevent episodes of bipolar disorder (Severus et al. 2014), and at least 48 studies (with 6,674 people) have found that lithium generally reduces the risk of suicide in people with mood disorders (Cipriani et al. 2013). One review of 37 trials (with 3,175 partici-

TABLE 8–1. Number of U.S. Food and Drug Administration
(FDA)–approved medications for selected major
mental illnesses (as of 2019)

Mental illness	Number of FDA-approved medications
Major depression	33
Schizophrenia	21
Bipolar disorder	14
Attention-deficit/hyperactivity disorder	9
Substance use disorders	8
Generalized anxiety disorder	7
Panic disorder	7
Obsessive-compulsive disorder	5
Posttraumatic stress disorder	2
Eating disorders	2

Note. Many other indicated medication treatments are supported by scientific data but
have not undergone the FDA approval process.

pants) found that *selective serotonin reuptake inhibitors* (SSRIs) were useful in
treating obsessive-compulsive disorder (OCD) (Skapinakis et al. 2016). A
recent meta-analysis found 167 studies (with 28,102 participants) showing
that *antipsychotics* help in treating schizophrenia (Leucht et al. 2017).

The evidence in favor of psychiatric medications is vast and represents
untold hours of effort by researchers and volunteer participants. Anyone
who needs such a medicine should feel should feel confident in going forward with this kind of medical treatment. But that does not mean that mental
health medications are instant cures. Some people have to try many different medications before finding one that works. Most people benefit, but
only a minority feel completely cured. In my experience as a psychiatrist,
people who only take a medicine and do nothing else for mental illness
seem to get partially better, but level off a long way from complete recovery.
And people who have trouble giving up bad habits like drinking too much
alcohol may not benefit much at all from a medication. On the other hand,
people who try multiple treatments (such as being more active, seeking social support, or getting talk therapy) typically improve the most, even if it
can take a long time to find success.

Treatment of mental illness is no different from the treatment of most other chronic medical conditions. Many people have to try a number of different medications for blood pressure before they find one that works well for them. And people who *only* take a medicine for diabetes or heart disease typically do not do as well as those who make positive lifestyle changes, such as diet and exercise, in addition to taking the medications.

Even when medicines are beneficial, all have risks, and all have downsides. There are no magic pills, as I like to remind myself. Aspirin, for example, is an over-the-counter medicine that is cheaply available. It is good for headaches and all manner of aches and pains. It is good for lowering fevers and for relieving arthritis. Aspirin is even good for helping to prevent heart attacks and strokes. Aspirin is a wonder drug, isn't it? Yes and no. Although aspirin is a wonderful medicine, it also has many risks. Aspirin can kill people in overdose. Some people have a toxic reaction and die even from normal doses of aspirin. Aspirin can cause ulcers or abnormal bleeding, especially in the gut. In addition to being dangerous, aspirin is not effective for everyone. Some people report that it works great for them, whereas others do not get much improvement from taking it.

The same applies for mental health medications: They are effective, but they also have risks and side effects. They can occasionally cause toxic reactions or put people at risk for other diseases. Some cause weight gain and a risk of diabetes, some interfere with sleep, and some can cause digestive problems. So how does a person decide whether to take a medication for mental health? *Generally, a person takes a medication when the benefits are likely to outweigh the risks.* For instance, if you do not have a mental illness, there is no benefit to be gained. This means that you would have only risks and side effects from taking a medicine, so you should not take it. However, because a mental illness can wreck your body or kill you (Chapter 6), it could make sense to take a medicine for mental illness, even if there are risks and side effects. Taking the medicine has risks, but not taking the medicine could have even more risks. So you might decide to put up with some side effects if they are far better than the toxic effects of your mental illness. The decision is similar to deciding whether to drive a car: Driving a car has big risks, including death, yet most people drive cars because the benefits outweigh the risks.

And though all medications have negative side effects, many people have not heard that there are some positive "side effects" for mental health treatments. Commonly used medications like lithium, antipsychotics, and antidepressants may slow the aging of cells, as assessed by longer telomere length (Bersani et al. 2015; see Chapter 6).(Bersani et al. 2015). Several psychiatric medications have been shown to promote the sprouting and growth of nerve cells, through a process known as neurogenesis. These include mood stabilizers (Jope and Nemeroff 2016; Monti et al. 2009), antidepressants (Schoenfeld and Cameron 2015), and newer antipsychotic medications (Chen and Nasrallah 2019). Lithium has been found to promote larger amounts of gray matter (nerve tissue) in the brain, at least for patients with bipolar disorder (Sun et al. 2018). Interestingly, SSRIs (and other medications that work on serotonin) seem to help prevent clotting and may lower the risk of heart attacks in individuals who are depressed (Andrade et al. 2013). The same medicines may also decrease important types of inflammation (Gałecki et al. 2018).

Many other biological treatments have scientific support for treating a variety of mental illnesses (Table 8–2). Some treatments are used for people who fail to benefit from the usual treatments. For example, vagus nerve stimulation (VNS) stimulates the brain through a major nerve in the neck, deep brain stimulation (DBS) uses tiny electrodes to stimulate places deep inside the brain (Khan et al. 2018), and ECT triggers seizure activity in the brain to treat severe and life-threatening symptoms (UK ECT Review Group 2003). Transcranial magnetic stimulation (TMS) uses powerful magnetic fields to stimulate the brain and treat OCD and major depression (Perera et al. 2016; Zhou et al. 2017). TMS may prove useful in the future for posttraumatic stress disorder (PTSD) and other disorders.

Many biological treatments are surprisingly simple. "Medical foods" such as methylfolate (a form of the vitamin B_9) and omega-3 fatty acids (fish oils) have been proven to help depression and other illnesses (Sarris et al. 2016). Diet may turn out to be an important factor in preventing mental illness for some individuals (Jacka 2017). Bright light therapy has been proven to help seasonal affective disorder, other mood disorders, and some sleep disorders (Penders et al. 2016; Van Maanen et al. 2016). Exercise can also benefit those with mental illness. Exercise causes the release of nerve growth factors that make neurons sprout and grow. In this way, it helps protect the brain against aging, improving sleep and cognitive function (Baumgart et al. 2015). Although exercise is not considered a stand-alone treatment for serious mental illness, it is proven to help depression, schizophrenia, and anxiety (Firth et al. 2015; Schuch et al. 2016; Stubbs et al. 2017). Exercise, even mild exercise, has powerful effects on the brain.

Psychological Treatments

The news is even better regarding the benefits of psychological treatments for mental illness. Psychotherapy (talk therapy) is real medical treatment and has been proven helpful for all major mental illnesses. Even disorders such as schizophrenia and bipolar disorder, once considered too "biological" for

TABLE 8–2. Biological treatments for mental illness (a partial list)

Psychiatric medications

Nonpsychiatric medications (e.g., thyroid hormone)

Vagus nerve stimulation (VNS)

Deep brain stimulation (DBS)

Electroconvulsive therapy (ECT)

Transcranial magnetic stimulation (TMS)

Medical foods (e.g., omega-3 fatty acids, methylfolate)

Diet

Bright light therapy

Exercise

talk therapy, have turned out to be responsive. So are difficult-to-treat conditions such as bulimia, social phobia, and borderline personality disorder. And numerous studies show that psychotherapy helps depression and anxiety.

Various types of cognitive therapy have been substantiated by scientific research (Table 8–3). Cognitive-behavioral therapy (CBT) is the most tested and best proven form of talk therapy. It involves understanding and changing distorted thoughts and perceptions. A 2006 review (Butler et al. 2006) identified 332 studies, and many more studies have been published since then (Hofmann et al. 2012). In fact, there is evidence that CBT is helpful for all the major mental health conditions, including mood disorders such as depression, psychotic disorders such as schizophrenia, and most anxiety disorders. It may be the best form of treatment available for bulimia and OCD.

Psychodynamic (insight-oriented) psychotherapy is also widely practiced. This kind of therapy involves the understanding of deeper patterns and motivations in our minds and relationships. It may be especially helpful for patients with depression, anxiety, and personality disorders. One rigorous review (Leichsenring et al. 2015) found 64 well-done studies showing the effectiveness of psychodynamic therapy for a range of psychiatric disorders (see also Abbass et al. 2014; Shedler 2010). There are many other types of talk therapy with good scientific support, including dialectal behavior therapy (DBT), interpersonal therapy (IPT), acceptance and commitment therapy (ACT), and motivational enhancement therapy (MET).

Talk therapy is medically powerful. It is proven to help a host of mental symptoms and illnesses, and the effect sizes have been comparable to those of psychiatric medications (Huhn et al. 2014). It shows efficacy for chronic

TABLE 8–3. Scientifically supported psychotherapies (a partial list)

Cognitive-behavioral therapy (CBT)

Psychodynamic insight-oriented psychotherapy

Interpersonal therapy (IPT)

Dialectical behavior therapy (DBT)

Mindfulness-based therapy (MBT)

Acceptance and commitment therapy (ACT)

Motivational interviewing (MI) and motivational enhancement therapy (MET)

Eye movement desensitization retraining and reprocessing (EMDR)

Source. American Psychological Association 2020.

pain, anger problems, and suicidality and other self-harm (Cristea et al. 2017; Henningsen et al. 2007). Psychotherapy is even superior to medication for some disorders such as OCD and specific phobia (Cuijpers et al. 2013b). We can also see evidence of its power in other scientific studies. Head scan studies have shown that psychotherapy changes the brain of those with mental illnesses, either back to normal patterns of activity or by activating new regions of the brain to aid in recovery (Barsaglini et al. 2014). Thus, there is no doubt that talk therapy changes the biology of the brain in important and powerful ways.

There is also evidence that psychotherapy has side benefits. Unlike medications, psychotherapy seems to help people even after they have stopped the treatment. It often helps prevent relapse to illness even after people have finished a course of treatment (Cuijpers et al. 2013a; Zhang et al. 2018). In some cases, people continue to improve for years after they have stopped therapy (Shedler 2010). Talk therapy helps reduce stress (Hofmann et al. 2012) and helps people function better and feel better generally (e.g., Kamenov et al. 2017; Laird et al. 2017). It also helps those with difficult-to-treat physical pain, fatigue, and other discomforts (Henningsen et al. 2007).

Talk therapy is now a well-documented medical treatment. However, when I was in medical training in the early 1990s, I was told we had a grand total of two well-performed medical studies on talk therapy. Two studies by themselves do not prove anything important in medicine. So at that time, no one could scientifically know whether talk therapy was psychobabble or real. Today we have thousands of studies and more than enough proof. In my opinion, this represents a silent revolution in medical science, one that few have noticed: Talking in a specific way (psychotherapy) profoundly changes our brains and bodies and is a powerful treatment for a long list of medical illnesses. This is a stunning development, one that proves there should be no conflict between psychology and biology in medicine.

The main downsides to talk therapy are the large investments of time and money involved. Psychotherapy takes a real commitment, and it often takes time to see results. Most of us find talk therapy to be anxiety-provoking, because it requires us to talk about painful experiences and admit to problems we wish we did not have. Finding the right therapy and the right therapist can also be a time-consuming and discouraging process. Although a majority of people find psychotherapy helpful, it is not a magical cure; a minority of people (5%–20%) report negative experiences or outcomes (Linden and Schermuly Haupt 2014).

There are numerous psychological therapies in addition to talk therapy (Table 8–4). Self-relaxation (Klainin-Yobas et al. 2015; Montero-Marin et al. 2018), biofeedback (Goessl et al. 2017), cognitive remediation (Wykes et al. 2011), computerized and smartphone-based psychotherapy (Firth et al. 2017a, 2017b), and guided self-help (Cuijpers et al. 2010) have proven effective for many people. Psychoeducation—simply learning about your illness and its treatment—has been proven to help outcomes in some cases (Donker et al. 2009; Lincoln et al. 2007).

Social Treatments

Biological and psychological treatments for mental illness make sense to most people, but some wonder how there could be social treatments for medical illness. Yet it turns out that social factors are profoundly important for both physical and mental health. For instance, good social support and connection actually decrease death rates and extend life. One review of 148 studies showed that social support is as good as quitting cigarettes, and better than exercise, for reducing risk of dying (Holt-Lunstad et al. 2010). Social support is also vital for resilience to mental illness. Social support makes people less likely to suffer from depression and anxiety (Cacioppo and Cacioppo 2014), and it makes a large difference when people have schizophrenia or bipolar disorder (Greenberg et al. 2014; Linz and Sturm 2013). Social support and activity even seem to decrease the risk of Alzheimer's dementia (Kuiper et al. 2015).

Fortunately, formal treatments are available that harness the power of social support (Table 8–5). Twelve-step programs such as Alcoholics Anonymous have led the way in showing us how a supportive group can make a decisive difference for the disease of addiction (Tonigan et al. 2018). NAMI (National Alliance on Mental Illness), Mental Health America, and other organizations offer support groups for people with mental health conditions and their family members. Group therapies are powerful for a range of mental illnesses, including DBT for borderline personality disor-

TABLE 8–4. Scientifically supported psychological treatments for mental illness (a partial list)

Psychotherapy (talk therapy)

Self-relaxation

Biofeedback

Cognitive remediation

Psychoeducation

Computerized and smartphone-based therapy

Guided self-help

Cognitive techniques

Mindfulness techniques

der (Cristea et al. 2017; Kösters et al. 2006). Family therapy can be especially helpful for schizophrenia (McFarlane 2016).

Many people also underestimate the power of hospital and residential treatment to calm severe psychiatric symptoms. Years ago when I was a psychiatric hospital orderly, I thought that it was only the medications that calmed symptoms in a remarkably quick time. Medicines do work for this purpose. But later I noticed that many people came into the psychiatric hospital, refused to take medicines, and still rapidly improved from psychosis and suicidality due to hospital treatment, which included regular sleep, a calm, low-stress environment, and supportive people (Katsakou and Priebe 2006). Even after a mental health crisis, most severely ill people benefit from group treatments such as residential care (living at a treatment center) or intensive outpatient treatment (several hours daily for 5 days a week) (Antonsen et al. 2014; Veale et al. 2016). Over the longer term, services like supported employment and Assertive Community Treatment (ACT) often make a massive positive difference. And early intervention services have the potential to alter the life course of those at risk for psychosis. If we (as a society) had the resources to offer long-term, intensive treatments such as these to people with severe mental illness, many more of the tragic cases we hear about today would have happier endings. Or so I believe based on personal experience.

Spiritual Treatments

If social treatments for mental illness sound a bit strange, what about spiritual ones? What would spiritual practices do for mental illness? Many people do not even believe that spirituality exists in any real sense, so how

TABLE 8–5.   Scientifically supported social treatments and activities (a partial list)

Group therapy (Kösters et al. 2006)

Family therapy (Claxton et al. 2017)

Social skills training (Kurtz and Mueser 2008; Wolstencroft et al. 2018)

Supported employment (Modini et al. 2016)

Assertive community treatment and early intervention services (Bond and Drake 2015; Correll et al. 2018)

Residential and intensive outpatient treatment (Antonsen et al. 2014; Veale et al. 2016)

Support groups and other peer support (Pfeiffer et al. 2011)

Alcoholics Anonymous and other twelve-step programs (Tonigan et al. 2018)

could it be relevant to the treatment of any medical illness? Yet according to scientific research, spirituality is an important factor in both physical and mental health, at least for people among those who are spiritually inclined. "Spirituality" here does not necessarily mean a belief in nonphysical realities. Rather, spirituality simply indicates an aspect of human nature, one we may express with or without supernatural beliefs. Spirituality allows us to experience the fact that we are part of something much greater than ourselves, that life has purpose and meaning beyond our individual existence, and that existence itself is fundamentally good.

What does spirituality have to do with health? Studies have shown that both religious and spiritual practices have a host of effects on your body and brain, most of them positive. For instance, there is evidence that meditation, spirituality, and religion decrease the normal shrinking of the brain (atrophy) that comes with age (Luders et al. 2015; Miller et al. 2014). Meditation also seems to cause greater telomere length (Schutte et al. 2020), indicating that it slows down this part of cellular aging (see Chapter 6). Meditation appears to lower inflammation, increase immunity, and lower stress hormones (Black and Slavich 2016). So does being religious (Shattuck and Muehlenbein 2020). Those who attend religious services also appear to live longer: A review of 69 long-term studies showed decreased death rates for those who attended regularly (Chida et al. 2009). And numerous studies have shown that mental health may also benefit: Religion and spirituality are associated with better coping with stress and less anxiety, depression, suicide, and substance abuse (Dew et al. 2008; Koenig 2009).

Because spiritual factors do affect health, these are being used in treating individuals with mental illness (Table 8–6). Specific therapies such as

TABLE 8–6. Spiritually related practices associated with mental health benefits

Meditation (Hilton et al. 2017)
Mindfulness (Goldberg et al. 2018)
Religious service attendance (Koenig 2009)
Prayer (Anderson and Nunnelley 2016)
Mantra repetition (Lynch et al. 2018)

mindfulness-based cognitive therapy (MBCT) and faith-adapted cognitive-behavioral therapy (F-CBT) have shown good results in studies so far (Anderson et al. 2015; Hofmann et al. 2012). Even outside of the office, practices such as meditation and mindfulness show benefit for conditions such as chronic pain, anxiety, and depression (Goldberg et al. 2018). Twelve-step programs like Alcoholics Anonymous ask people to turn their lives to a "power greater than themselves" for relief of addiction. Some studies have shown that prayer also may be helpful for alcohol use disorders and major depression (Anderson and Nunnelley 2016). Others have shown that mantra repetition (repeating a word or phrase from your spiritual tradition) can help conditions such as PTSD and anxiety (Lynch et al. 2018).

The Bottom Line

We have many treatments to offer to individuals with mental illness. We have more treatments than I could possibly discuss in a book of this sort, and all of them have a real scientific basis. Every person is different, and everyone with a mental health condition will need a different set of treatments. Usually, people do best with a range for treatments, from biological to psychological to social and spiritual. Finding just the right mix of treatments can be a long and grueling process, but in my experience, people who do not die or give up eventually find what they need. Many must endure years of discouragement and doubt along the way, grappling with the fear that nothing will ever work. But eventually, most people who do not give up get a handle on their symptoms and find a way to make treatment work. Gradually and unpredictably, they begin to move from impairment to recovery. They begin to rebuild their lives, not as life would have been without mental illness, but in a new and unforeseeable way. Anyone who has ever experienced this kind of "turnaround" should count themselves lucky. I have been fortunate enough to see it many times and am in awe of those who have made the journey. In the next chapter, I want to share a little bit of their wisdom and experience.

Advice for Advocacy

- Laypersons can find the distinction between acute and chronic illness to be strange at first, but it is often worth the investment of time to help them understand.
- If time does not allow a discussion of acute vs. chronic illness, you can compare mental health conditions with other important medical problems, including high blood pressure, heart disease, and diabetes. Virtually everyone can relate to these examples.
- If you are a psychiatrist or other medical doctor, people might assume that you mean "medications" when you say "treatment." You will have to make an effort to emphasize other types of treatments. Similarly, if you are a psychotherapist, you may need to mention medications specifically. Either way, interdisciplinary "turf battles" are out of place in the context of advocacy.
- Some mental health professionals may be uncomfortable discussing spiritual and religious factors in recovery. If you feel this way, keep in mind that most people identify themselves as spiritual or religious, and many assume that mental health practitioners will be hostile to their religion. On the basis of science, you can affirm health-promoting spiritual and religious practices without endorsing any specific forms of spirituality or religion.
- Emphasizing the good news about treatment is critical for advocacy. At the same time, remember that there are many suicide survivors and people dealing with treatment-resistant forms of illness. These individuals may begin to feel guilty or inadequate when you emphasize successful treatments, so make an effort to reassure them that they are not failing in any way. As usual, the best way is to compare mental health treatment with other forms of medical treatment. Tragically, regardless of treatment, there will always be treatment-resistant and even fatal cases.

References

Abbass AA, Kisely SR, Town JM, et al: Short-term psychodynamic psychotherapies for common mental disorders. Cochrane Database Syst Rev (7):CD004687, 2014

Abdollahi A, LeBouthillier DM, Najafi M, et al: Effect of exercise augmentation of cognitive behavioural therapy for the treatment of suicidal ideation and depression. J Affect Disord 219:58–63, 2017

American Psychological Association: Psychological treatments. Society of Clinical Psychology, Division 12, American Psychological Association, 2020. Available at: www.div12.org/treatments/. Accessed August 3, 2020.

Anderson JW, Nunnelley PA: Private prayer associations with depression, anxiety and other health conditions: an analytical review of clinical studies. Postgrad Med 128(7):635–641, 2016

Anderson N, Heywood-Everett S, Siddiqi N, et al: Faith-adapted psychological therapies for depression and anxiety: systematic review and meta-analysis. J Affect Disord 176:183–196, 2015

Andrade C, Kumar C, Surya S: Cardiovascular mechanisms of SSRI drugs and their benefits and risks in ischemic heart disease and heart failure. Int Clin Psychopharmacol 28(3):145–155, 2013

Antonsen BT, Klungsøyr O, Kamps A, et al: Step-down versus outpatient psychotherapeutic treatment for personality disorders: 6-year follow-up of the Ullevål Personality Project. BMC Psychiatry 14:119, 2014

Barsaglini A, Sartori G, Benetti S, et al: The effects of psychotherapy on brain function: a systematic and critical review. Prog Neurobiol 114:1–14, 2014

Bauer UE, Briss PA, Goodman RA, et al: Prevention of chronic disease in the 21st century: elimination of the leading preventable causes of premature death and disability in the USA. Lancet 384(9937):45–52, 2014

Baumgart M, Snyder HM, Carrillo MC, et al: Summary of the evidence on modifiable risk factors for cognitive decline and dementia: a population-based perspective. Alzheimers Dement 11(6):718–726, 2015

Bersani FS, Lindqvist D, Mellon SH, et al: Telomerase activation as a possible mechanism of action for psychopharmacological interventions. Drug Discov Today 20(11):1305–1309, 2015

Black DS, Slavich GM: Mindfulness meditation and the immune system: a systematic review of randomized controlled trials. Ann NY Acad Sci 1373(1):13–24, 2016

Bond GR, Drake RE: The critical ingredients of assertive community treatment. World Psychiatry 14(2):240–242, 2015

Butler AC, Chapman JE, Forman EM, et al: The empirical status of cognitive-behavioral therapy: a review of meta-analyses. Clin Psychol Rev 26(1):17–31, 2006

Buttorff C, Ruder T, Bauman M: Multiple Chronic Conditions in the United States. Santa Monica, CA, RAND, 2017

Cacioppo JT, Cacioppo S: Social relationships and health: the toxic effects of perceived social isolation. Soc Personal Psychol Compass 8(2):58–72, 2014

Centers for Disease Control and Prevention: National Ambulatory Care Survey Summary: 2016 National Summary Tables. 2016. Available at: www.cdc.gov/nchs/data/ahcd/namcs_summary/2016_namcs_web_tables.pdf. Accessed August 3, 2020.

Chen AT, Nasrallah HA: Neuroprotective effects of the second generation antipsychotics. Schizophr Res 208:1–7, 2019

Chida Y, Steptoe A, Powell LH: Religiosity/spirituality and mortality: a systematic quantitative review. Psychother Psychosom 78(2):81–90, 2009

Cipriani A, Hawton K, Stockton S, et al: Lithium in the prevention of suicide in mood disorders: updated systematic review and meta-analysis. BMJ 346:f3646, 2013

Cipriani A, Furukawa TA, Salanti G, et al: Comparative efficacy and acceptability of 21 antidepressant drugs for the acute treatment of adults with major depressive disorder: a systematic review and network meta-analysis. Lancet 391(10128):1357–1366, 2018

Claxton M, Onwumere J, Fornells-Ambrojo M: Do family interventions improve outcomes in early psychosis? A systematic review and meta-analysis. Front Psychol 8:371, 2017

Correll CU, Galling B, Pawar A, et al: Comparison of early intervention services vs treatment as usual for early phase psychosis: a systematic review, meta-analysis, and meta-regression. JAMA Psychiatry 75(6):555–565, 2018

Cristea IA, Gentili C, Cotet CD, et al: Efficacy of psychotherapies for borderline personality disorder: a systematic review and meta-analysis. JAMA Psychiatry 74(4):319–328, 2017

Cuijpers P, Donker T, van Straten A, et al: Is guided self-help as effective as face-to-face psychotherapy for depression and anxiety disorders? A systematic review and meta-analysis of comparative outcome studies. Psychol Med 40(12):1943–1957, 2010

Cuijpers P, Hollon SD, van Straten A, et al: Does cognitive behaviour therapy have an enduring effect that is superior to keeping patients on continuation pharmacotherapy? A meta-analysis. BMJ Open 3(4):e002542, 2013a

Cuijpers P, Sijbrandij M, Koole SL, et al: The efficacy of psychotherapy and pharmacotherapy in treating depressive and anxiety disorders: a meta-analysis of direct comparisons. World Psychiatry 12(2):137–148, 2013b

Dew RE, Daniel SS, Armstrong TD, et al: Religion/spirituality and adolescent psychiatric symptoms: a review. Child Psychiatry Hum Dev 39(4):381–398, 2008

Donker T, Griffiths KM, Cuijpers P, et al: Psychoeducation for depression, anxiety and psychological distress: a meta-analysis. BMC Med 7(1):79, 2009

Firth J, Cotter J, Elliott R, et al: A systematic review and meta-analysis of exercise interventions in schizophrenia patients. Psychol Med 45(7):1343–1361, 2015

Firth J, Torous J, Nicholas J, et al: Can smartphone mental health interventions reduce symptoms of anxiety? A meta-analysis of randomized controlled trials. J Affect Disord 218:15–22, 2017a

Firth J, Torous J, Nicholas J, et al: The efficacy of smartphone-based mental health interventions for depressive symptoms: a meta-analysis of randomized controlled trials. World Psychiatry 16(3):287–298, 2017b

Gałecki P, Mossakowska-Wojcik J, Talarowska M: The anti-inflammatory mechanism of antidepressants—SSRIs, SNRIs. Prog Neuropsychopharmacol Biol Psychiatry 80:291–294, 2018

Goessl VC, Curtiss JE, Hofmann SG: The effect of heart rate variability biofeedback training on stress and anxiety: a meta-analysis. Psychol Med 47(15):2578–2586, 2017

Goldberg SB, Tucker RP, Greene PA, et al: Mindfulness-based interventions for psychiatric disorders: a systematic review and meta-analysis. Clin Psychol Rev 59:52–60, 2018

Greenberg S, Rosenblum KL, McInnis MG, et al: The role of social relationships in bipolar disorder: a review. Psychiatry Res 219(2):248–254, 2014

Harrington A: Mind Fixers: Psychiatry's Troubled Search for the Biology of Mental Illness. New York, WW Norton, 2019

Henningsen P, Zipfel S, Herzog W: Management of functional somatic syndromes. Lancet 369(9565):946–955, 2007

Hilton L, Maher AR, Colaiaco B, et al: Meditation for posttraumatic stress: systematic review and meta-analysis. Psychol Trauma 9(4):453–460, 2017

Hofmann SG, Asnaani A, Vonk IJ, et al: The efficacy of cognitive behavioral therapy: a review of meta-analyses. Cognit Ther Res 36(5):427–440, 2012

Holt-Lunstad J, Smith TB, Layton JB: Social relationships and mortality risk: a meta-analytic review. PLoS Med 7(7):e1000316, 2010

Huhn M, Tardy M, Spineli LM, et al: Efficacy of pharmacotherapy and psychotherapy for adult psychiatric disorders: a systematic overview of meta-analyses. JAMA Psychiatry 71(6):706–715, 2014

Jacka FN: Nutritional psychiatry: where to next? EBioMedicine 17:24–29, 2017

Jope RS, Nemeroff CB: Lithium to the rescue. Cerebrum 2016:cer-02-16, 2016

Kamenov K, Twomey C, Cabello M, et al: The efficacy of psychotherapy, pharmacotherapy and their combination on functioning and quality of life in depression: a meta-analysis. Psychol Med 47(3):414–425, 2017

Katsakou C, Priebe S: Outcomes of involuntary hospital admission—a review. Acta Psychiatr Scand 114(4):232–241, 2006

Khan AM, Ahmed R, Kotapati VP, et al: Vagus nerve stimulation (VNS) vs. deep brain stimulation (DBS) treatment for major depressive disorder and bipolar depression: a comparative meta-analytic review. Int J Med Public Health 8(3):119–130, 2018

Klainin-Yobas P, Oo WN, Suzanne Yew PY, et al: Effects of relaxation interventions on depression and anxiety among older adults: a systematic review. Aging Ment Health 19(12):1043–1055, 2015

Koenig HG: Religion and medicine I: historical background and reasons for separation. Int J Psychiatry Med 30(4):385–398, 2000

Koenig HG: Research on religion, spirituality, and mental health: a review. Can J Psychiatry 54(5):283–291, 2009

Kösters M, Burlingame GM, Nachtigall C, et al: A meta-analytic review of the effectiveness of inpatient group psychotherapy. Group Dynamics: Theory, Research, and Practice 10(2):146–163, 2006

Kuiper JS, Zuidersma M, Voshaar RC, et al: Social relationships and risk of dementia: a systematic review and meta-analysis of longitudinal cohort studies. Ageing Res Rev 22:39–57, 2015

Kurtz MM, Mueser KT: A meta-analysis of controlled research on social skills training for schizophrenia. J Consult Clin Psychol 76(3):491–504, 2008

Laing RD: The Divided Self: An Existential Study in Sanity and Madness. Harmondsworth, UK, Penguin, 1965

Laird KT, Tanner-Smith EE, Russell AC, et al: Comparative efficacy of psychological therapies for improving mental health and daily functioning in irritable bowel syndrome: a systematic review and meta-analysis. Clin Psychol Rev 51:142–152, 2017

Leichsenring F, Luyten P, Hilsenroth MJ, et al: Psychodynamic therapy meets evidence-based medicine: a systematic review using updated criteria. Lancet Psychiatry 2(7):648–660, 2015

Leucht S, Hierl S, Kissling W, et al: Putting the efficacy of psychiatric and general medicine medication into perspective: review of meta-analyses. Br J Psychiatry 200(2):97–106, 2012

Leucht S, Leucht C, Huhn M, et al: Sixty years of placebo-controlled antipsychotic drug trials in acute schizophrenia: systematic review, Bayesian meta-analysis, and meta-regression of efficacy predictors. Am J Psychiatry 174(10):927–942, 2017

Lincoln TM, Wilhelm K, Nestoriuc Y: Effectiveness of psychoeducation for relapse, symptoms, knowledge, adherence and functioning in psychotic disorders: a meta-analysis. Schizophr Res 96(1–3):232–245, 2007

Linden M, Schermuly Haupt ML: Definition, assessment and rate of psychotherapy side effects. World Psychiatry 13(3):306–309, 2014

Linz SJ, Sturm BA: The phenomenon of social isolation in the severely mentally ill. Perspect Psychiatr Care 49(4):243–254, 2013

Luders E, Cherbuin N, Kurth F: Forever Young(er): potential age-defying effects of long-term meditation on gray matter atrophy. Front Psychol 5:1551, 2015

Luhrmann TM: Of Two Minds: An Anthropologist Looks at American Psychiatry. New York, Vintage, 2001

Lynch J, Prihodova L, Dunne PJ, et al: Mantra meditation for mental health in the general population: a systematic review. Eur J Integr Med 23:101–108, 2018

McFarlane WR: Family interventions for schizophrenia and the psychoses: a review. Fam Process 55(3):460–482, 2016

Miller L, Bansal R, Wickramaratne P, et al: Neuroanatomical correlates of religiosity and spirituality: a study in adults at high and low familial risk for depression. JAMA Psychiatry 71(2):128–135, 2014

Modini M, Tan L, Brinchmann B, et al: Supported employment for people with severe mental illness: systematic review and meta-analysis of the international evidence. Br J Psychiatry 209(1):14–22, 2016

Montero-Marin J, Garcia-Campayo J, López-Montoyo A, et al: Is cognitive-behavioural therapy more effective than relaxation therapy in the treatment of anxiety disorders? A meta-analysis. Psychol Med 48(9):1427–1436, 2018

Monti B, Polazzi E, Contestabile A: Biochemical, molecular and epigenetic mechanisms of valproic acid neuroprotection. Curr Mol Pharmacol 2(1):95–109, 2009

Penders TM, Stanciu CN, Schoemann AM, et al: Bright light therapy as augmentation of pharmacotherapy for treatment of depression: a systematic review and meta-analysis. Prim Care Companion CNS Disord 18(5), 2016

Perera T, George MS, Grammer G, et al: The clinical TMS society consensus review and treatment recommendations for TMS therapy for major depressive disorder. Brain Stimul 9(3):336–346, 2016

Pfeiffer PN, Heisler M, Piette JD, et al: Efficacy of peer support interventions for depression: a meta-analysis. Gen Hosp Psychiatry 33(1):29–36, 2011

Sarris J, Murphy J, Mischoulon D, et al: Adjunctive nutraceuticals for depression: a systematic review and meta-analyses. Am J Psychiatry 173(6):575–587, 2016

Scheff TJ: Being Mentally Ill: A Sociological Theory. Chicago, IL, Aldine, 1966

Schoenfeld TJ, Cameron HA: Adult neurogenesis and mental illness. Neuropsychopharmacology 40(1):113–128, 2015

Schuch FB, Vancampfort D, Richards J, et al: Exercise as a treatment for depression: a meta-analysis adjusting for publication bias. J Psychiatr Res 77:42–51, 2016

Schutte NS, Malouff JM, Keng SL: Meditation and telomere length: a meta-analysis. Psychol Health 35(8):901–915, 2020

Severus E, Taylor MJ, Sauer C, et al: Lithium for prevention of mood episodes in bipolar disorders: systematic review and meta-analysis. Int J Bipolar Disord 2(1):15, 2014

Shattuck EC, Muehlenbein MP: Religiosity/spirituality and physiological markers of health. J Relig Health 59(2):1035–1054, 2020

Shedler J: The efficacy of psychodynamic psychotherapy. Am Psychol 65(2):98–109, 2010

Skapinakis P, Caldwell DM, Hollingworth W, et al: Pharmacological and psychotherapeutic interventions for management of obsessive-compulsive disorder in adults: a systematic review and network meta-analysis. Lancet Psychiatry 3(8):730–739, 2016

Stanford MS: Grace for the Afflicted: A Clinical and Biblical Perspective on Mental Illness. Downers Grove, IL, InterVarsity Press, 2012

Stubbs B, Vancampfort D, Rosenbaum S, et al: An examination of the anxiolytic effects of exercise for people with anxiety and stress-related disorders: a meta-analysis. Psychiatry Res 249:102–108, 2017

Sun YR, Herrmann N, Scott CJ, et al: Global grey matter volume in adult bipolar patients with and without lithium treatment: a meta-analysis. J Affect Disord 225:599–606, 2018

Tonigan JS, Pearson MR, Magill M, et al: AA attendance and abstinence for dually diagnosed patients: a meta-analytic review. Addiction 113(11):1970–1981, 2018

UK ECT Review Group: Efficacy and safety of electroconvulsive therapy in depressive disorders: a systematic review and meta-analysis. Lancet 361(9360):799–808, 2003

Van Maanen A, Meijer AM, van der Heijden KB, et al: The effects of light therapy on sleep problems: a systematic review and meta-analysis. Sleep Med Rev 29:52–62, 2016

Veale D, Naismith I, Miles S, et al: Outcomes for residential or inpatient intensive treatment of obsessive-compulsive disorder: a systematic review and meta-analysis. J Obsessive-Compuls Relat Disord 8:38–49, 2016

Wolstencroft J, Robinson L, Srinivasan R, et al: A systematic review of group social skills interventions, and meta-analysis of outcomes, for children with high functioning ASD. J Autism Dev Disord 48(7):2293–2307, 2018

Wykes T, Huddy V, Cellard C, et al: A meta-analysis of cognitive remediation for schizophrenia: methodology and effect sizes. Am J Psychiatry 168(5):472–485, 2011

Zhang Z, Zhang L, Zhang G, et al: The effect of CBT and its modifications for relapse prevention in major depressive disorder: a systematic review and meta-analysis. BMC Psychiatry 18(1):50, 2018

Zhou DD, Wang W, Wang GM, et al: An updated meta-analysis: short-term therapeutic effects of repeated transcranial magnetic stimulation in treating obsessive-compulsive disorder. J Affect Disord 215:187–196, 2017

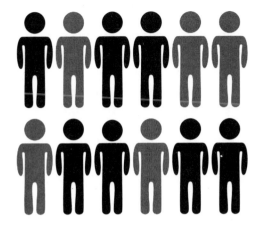

Mental Illness Is Our Teacher

Half Truth: Serious mental illness exerts a devastating effect on the lives of those who have it.

Whole Truth: Even those with the most severe types of mental illness can find recovery and develop a deep wisdom about life in the process.

Important Points

- People with mental illness are no different from anyone else. Everyone gets sick, and mental illness is one form of getting sick.
- On average, mental illness begins around age 14. Because mental illness begins earlier than most chronic illnesses, people with mental illness are pushed to learn about life and mature at a younger age than most.
- Acceptance is the key to recovery from mental illness, and the key to living life well. *Acceptance* does not mean approval or despair. It means taking life on its own terms.

- Acceptance leads to recovery. *Recovery* does not mean cure or unlimited success. It means making a good, meaningful life within the limitations of life, including illness.

- People who have been through their own process of recovery have much to teach the rest of us about life. We should listen to them and learn from their wisdom.

Introduction

For mental health professionals, there is an obvious danger to talking about mental illness from a scientific and objective viewpoint: People with mental illness may sound like anonymous and passive recipients of treatments performed by knowledgeable and implicitly superior professionals. Nothing could be further from the truth, however. Good clinicians have always recognized that the therapeutic alliance is the sine qua non of all effective treatment. And a good therapeutic alliance involves not only a sense of partnership and respect but a recognition that the patient is responsible for the lion's share of treatment. In other words, the patient is in the driver's seat of his or her own life, and we professionals are at best merely passengers who attempt to help navigate. We do have expertise and power in the treatment relationship, but successful treatment requires that we play "second fiddle" to the patient's melody.

More deeply, the difference between a patient and a professional is a difference of social role and nothing else. We are not professionals because we are superior, because we have figured out life, or because we are not subject to mental illnesses. We too suffer from mental illnesses; we too have problems and struggles; we too become overwhelmed, baffled, and confused by life. And although we do not discuss such personal experiences in our professional roles, we should never lose sight of them. Illnesses, problems, and struggles are simply part of the human condition.

Individuals who cope with mental illness do not dwell in a static and permanent sick role of passivity and disability. Those who pursue recovery are not simply survivors. They are fellow human beings who have summoned the courage to walk the same path we all face, the path through adversity, illness, and limitation. Their recovery work is both admirable and directly relatable to the deepest challenges that all of us will face in life. Everyone who seeks a good and meaningful life must do so in the presence of limitation and suffering, and those who do so in the presence of mental illness can attain the deepest success available in life. If we cannot clearly convey this truth in our work as advocates, we will not alter the diffuse public perception of people with mental illness as inferior, pitiful, and fundamentally other.

Mental Illness: Those People or Us People?

I hope that the answer to this question has been clear from the first chapter of this book, and I hope that the answer now seems as obvious to you as it does to me. Mental illness is not about those people, but about us people. Mental illness affects us all. We have had it, or we love someone who has had it. If we have not had it, there is a good chance that we will experience it at some time in life. And even if we never have it ourselves, we are no different from people who do have it. On a deeper level, it really doesn't matter whether we will ever experience mental illness ourselves. For it is certain that we will all get sick at some point in life, and mental illness is just another way that human beings get sick. Mental illness is not fundamentally different from heart disease or cancer or all the other ways that people get sick. Getting sick is part of being human, and everyone gets sick. Usually, the illness is mild or temporary. But sometimes we get seriously and chronically ill. If we live long enough, this will be part of life.

People with mental illness are just normal people who have mental illness. They are not a breed apart. They feel like you would feel if you had the same symptoms. Imagine how you would feel if you were in the worst mood of your life, then woke up the next day feeling even worse (depression). Imagine if you were so nervous that you could not sleep at night or focus to do your job in the day; then imagine that nothing you did to calm yourself down would work (generalized anxiety). Imagine how you would feel if you started hearing voices—not imaginary ones, but real, objective and distracting voices outside of yourself (schizophrenia).

You would probably feel the same shock, horror, and shame that most people experience with mental illness. You would be appalled at your inability to push through, your inability to control your own mind and behaviors. You might have the feeling of being in a dream—of doing things that are out of character and embarrassing, yet not being able to stop yourself from doing them. It would probably take you a long time to realize that you were having an illness, and that there was no way to control your symptoms simply with willpower. It would take even longer to admit this to yourself, and longer still to begin to seek help. Yet seeking help would only be the beginning. You would just be at the beginning of a long struggle with mental illness.

As a psychiatrist, I often get calls from people seeking help for mental illness. Whenever I do, I remind myself that the person calling me is already worn down by the task of dealing with such an illness. By the time you call some stranger for help with mental illness, you will have already done every single thing you know to make yourself feel better. In all probability, you may have already searched online, already tried self-help books and over-the-counter cures. You may have already asked family members or close friends for help. Maybe you have talked with your family doctor about your options. But the last thing you want to do is to take the risk of calling someone you do not know, some therapist or psychiatrist who might or might not be right for you. Even when you are willing to reach out, it is difficult to find the right therapist, or maybe even any available psychiatrist. There is a nationwide shortage of psychiatrists, and although there are many more psychotherapists, getting insurance coverage for good treatment is not easy. Neither is figuring out how to get child care or time off from work for your appointments. And all of these complications occur before people even start treatment, before they begin the daunting process of recovery.

No serious illness is easy. Feeling guilty, ashamed, and weak for being sick cuts across both mental and other physical illnesses. And all serious illnesses bring suffering on top of shame, disability on top of self-doubt. Significant illness is scary, unsettling, and disruptive to the routine of normal life. It takes away our ability to function normally and be independent. It is usually painful. It is always frustrating and daunting.

How does having mental illness compare with having other illnesses? Like most other kinds of illness, mental illness can be mild, moderate, or severe. So we have to compare like for like, not severe mental illness with some other mild physical illness (such as a cold). People who have had both severe mental illness and other severe illnesses tell me that the experience of mental illness is worse. Certainly, more stigma and shame are associated with mental illness. The struggle to get treatment and to get coverage for treatment is greater. The levels of disability and death are equally as bad. But the pain is worse. People who have had severe physical pain (such as during childbirth or from kidney stones or broken bones) tell me repeatedly that the pain of mental illness is worse. And I know people who have been wounded in battle and who have had severe injuries from car accidents who say that mental illness is more painful. They should know.

Meeting Mental Illness: Pity or Empathy?

When I talk to people dealing with mental illness, I do not feel sorry for them. I do not feel depressed by them. And I do not feel impatient with them. Instead, I admire them, I respect them, and I feel inspired by them. For me, talking with someone who has mental illness is like talking to someone who has been through combat. I certainly do not envy them. I hope that I never have to go through such a battle myself and that I never have to endure what they have endured. But I feel a sense of awe and a deep respect for anyone who could face such an experience and survive, much less somehow function in the midst of it. And I want to know how they did it. How could they get through all that and go on? No one gets a medal for getting through mental illness. But everyone who does get through it should get a medal, and so should the family that supports them. In many ways, getting through mental illness is as bad and overwhelming an experience as going off to war. People who have been to war have told me so.

Like people who go into combat (Figure 9–1), people dealing with significant mental illness cannot be sure they will survive. Some make it, but others—friends and fellow soldiers—don't. Many more are wounded, and need treatment and rehabilitation to function again. Everyone who goes through combat is terrified and wishes they did not have to be there. And when things are at their worst, the only thing to do is to hunker down and try to survive. Some days, the person just wants to survive, just live to fight another day. Some days, survival alone is a massive accomplishment. The person just wants to survive and somehow make it "home" alive, make it back to normal life.

Like war, mental illness leaves no one unchanged. People have wounds and scars that they will carry for the rest of their lives. They will never be the same. They will always have regret, guilt, and sadness, whether or not they deserve to. They will have experiences they cannot fully put into words. They will have trouble explaining what mental illness was like to people who have never been through it. They will envy people who have never had to experience the same thing and will never know what it is like.

Mental illness gives people a kind of knowledge they did not want, and a kind of wisdom they wish they never needed. But it is a kind of wisdom the rest of us will eventually need. Most of us will eventually get sick with serious illness. And people with mental illness have a lot to teach us about how to deal with such universal human experiences.

Learning to Live With Life

As a psychiatry trainee at an internationally known center for psychiatry, I often found myself in a strange situation. I was learning the ropes and happy to be doing so at a first-class institution. People came from all over the country and all over the world for treatment. And that was just the problem. Who was I to cure them? What was I, a trainee, supposed to do about their illnesses? People would say things like "I've tried all the local psychiatrists and doctors in my area. I've tried the hospitals. I have tried every

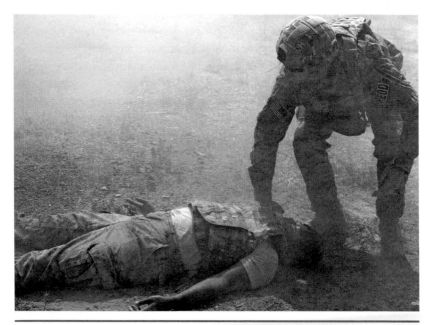

FIGURE 9–1. The trauma of war.

Source. United States Air Force (USAF). "EOD Receives Tactical Combat Training." April 31. 2017. Photo by Chase Cannon. Available at: www.12af.acc.af.mil/News/Photos/igphoto/2001758234. Retrieved November 19, 2019.

medicine and read every self-help book. Nothing has worked, but I knew if I could just get myself here, just make it to this place, you could help me!" Gulp. How was I supposed to know more than all these other doctors and therapists and writers of self-help books? I was just learning myself!

Because of this dilemma, I developed a habit in my work. I started asking the patients what helped them. There were many people who had come for treatment and stayed long-term, settling into the local community. There were people who had severe, life-threatening, and treatment-resistant illness who somehow got better. These included people who had tried to kill themselves multiple times, who were addicted to dangerous substances, who refused to take their medicines, who got violent, or who just could not seem to find anything that worked. So how did they do it? How did they survive and get better?

I asked every single person that I met, "How did you do it? How did you get better?" To my surprise, their answers were very similar. They were not identical, not word for word. So this wasn't something people just heard repeatedly and parroted back. Everyone had their own individual version, but it always went something like this: They would start with a long pause, a sigh, and a faraway look, and then say something like this:

Well, for a long time I just did not want to have the illness. I tried to act like I was fine, like I could party, take drugs, overwork, and stay out as late as I wanted. I would skip appointments and throw away medicines. I tried not to be sick. But when I acted like that, things would just go from bad to worse. I would wind up in bed for weeks, unemployed, suicidal, and eventually in the hospital. I hated the thought of having an illness, but eventually I got to the point that I could not deny it anymore. Eventually, I had to admit that I don't want this illness, but I have it. I hate the idea of being sick, but I'm sick. And I am just going to have to learn to live with this. Somehow, I am going to have to live a life with the illness. I have to admit it and accept it. And from that point on, the moment I accepted it, things started to get better. They weren't perfect and they weren't great, but they gradually got better and better.

As more and more people said the same thing, I was stunned. I thought everybody would have a different "secret" to treatment success, and that I would have a list of lots of things that might work. I thought people would say they found just the right medicine, or just the right kind of therapy. I thought they might tell me about some amazing self-help book or treatment program. They did benefit from all of those things, but none of them said the specific treatments were decisive. They all said that there was one thing that made the critical difference: acceptance.

What Is Acceptance?

I thought a long time about these answers. I tried to wrap my mind around what must have happened. I mean, wasn't it obvious to these people that they had an illness from the time it started to get bad? Didn't the doctor tell them their diagnosis? Didn't they know why they were supposed to take the medicine or go to appointments? Obviously they knew. They knew, but at first they only knew intellectually. They did not know emotionally or practically. They did not know and accept their illness at deeper levels, at the heart level and gut level. They knew they were sick but tried to live as if they weren't, think as if they weren't, and feel as if they weren't. And they hit the wall over and over, until they finally came to acceptance.

What is acceptance? Acceptance is not approval. Acceptance is not saying, "I'm so glad I got this illness that changed my life forever." Acceptance is not giving up. Acceptance is not saying, "I'm sick and there is nothing I can do about it. I give up." And acceptance is not identifying with the illness. Acceptance is not saying, "I'm just a schizophrenic," or, "I'm just an addict." Acceptance is simply taking reality as it is and learning to live with it. Acceptance is admitting, "I have problems, I have imperfections, I have a chronic illness. I am so much more than an illness, but I have to go on with this illness, because I will not be able to go on any other way."

The Paradox of Self-Improvement

Twelve-step programs such as Alcoholics Anonymous have led the way in teaching people how to live with mental illnesses. Twelve-step groups ask people to admit that they have an illness and to admit that they cannot control it. The first step is acceptance: "We admitted that we were powerless over alcohol and our lives had become unmanageable" (Alcoholics Anonymous 2001). The second step involves a willingness to seek a "power greater than myself," some outside source of help.

Strange to say, *the first step of making yourself better is to admit that you cannot make yourself better. And the only way to change yourself is to accept yourself the way you are, problems and all.* I call this the paradox of self-improvement. There are lots of problems in life that we can solve, and all of us go forward with solving them on a daily basis. But there are some that we cannot solve, no matter how hard we try to control them. Illness, by definition, is not something we can control by willpower or trying harder. No matter how hard we try, things just will not work. For instance, no matter how hard people with severe depression try to get up and function, they will not be able to function normally. No matter how hard people with schizophrenia try to focus, they will not be able to focus as well as they once did. Therefore, people with a mental illness have to accept that they cannot control the illness. They cannot make it go away and they cannot suppress the symptoms. They have to learn to live with it and accept treatment.

Strangely enough, the best way to change is to admit we cannot make ourselves change. The best way to deal with a problem is to admit we have the problem. The only way we can get better from having an illness is to admit that we have the illness whether we want it or not. The more we can look in the mirror and say, "I accept you just the way you are, right now, with no reservations," the more we will find ourselves in a process of healing and growth.

The Great American Myth

Everybody knows about acceptance, but it is generally not the way most people approach self-help. Most self-help best sellers promise a lot: to take away worry, cure our illnesses (usually without drugs), organize us, help us enjoy life, and make us happy. If all they did was say, "Accept your problems," they would be short books, and no one would read them anyway. Most self-help books and self-help gurus work within what I call the Great

American Myth. The Great American Myth goes like this: "If you want it bad enough and you work hard enough, you can do anything." And the Great American Myth is true, to a degree. I do not call it a myth because it is untrue. I call it a myth because it is a story that tells us something deep about life. We read autobiographies and best sellers that tell stories of people who illustrate the Great American Myth, including Abraham Lincoln and Barack Obama, who went from obscurity to becoming president. We hear about sports stars, such as quarterback Kurt Warner, who was stocking groceries one year and winning the Super Bowl the next year. We watch unknown amateur performers turn into superstars after appearing on television shows such as *American Idol*. And in movies such as *Rocky* and *The Blind Side*, we watch heroes who had nothing somehow overcome everything with courage and grit. Everybody loves a winner, and everybody likes stories such as these.

The best part about the Great American Myth is that it inspires us. All of us have hopes and dreams, and the Great American Myth tells us not to give up on our hopes and dreams. It tells us that maybe we, ordinary people, can do extraordinary things. Maybe we can be more than we ever thought possible. Maybe we can come from nothing and become somethings. Yes, there is great truth in this myth, and much good has resulted from it.

However, there is also a downside to this myth. The Great American Myth tells us that we can do anything, as long as we work hard enough and want it badly enough. Well, what if I tried to do something and did not succeed? What if I tried repeatedly yet failed to accomplish my goal? What if I wanted to be president, but never became president? What if I wanted to be an NFL quarterback, but had a career-ending injury in high school? The Great American Myth implies that I did not work hard enough or want it badly enough. If I did not realize my dream, it must be my fault. I must be a failure. And even if nobody ever tells me this, I am going to feel like a failure inside, because my dreams did not come true.

Myth and Reality

There is a reality greater than the Great American Myth. The reality is that if your dream is to become president of the United States, you probably will not succeed. There are over 320 million Americans, but there can only be so many presidents, one or so every 4–8 years. And there are also limits to the numbers of Olympic gold medalists, movie stars, and lots of other things people dream about becoming.

In truth, some of our dreams come true, but most do not. One of mine was to be a running back in the NFL. Another was to be a jazz musician. It turns out that I have genetics for being average athletically and a bit above average musically. Even if I could have worked with NFL coaches from infancy, I never would have become an NFL running back. I could have practiced endlessly and never become a professional musician. I did not have the genetic makeup to do these things, or to become president, or to be a successful actor. And there is no shame in this. The reality is that all of us have different collections of abilities, and all of us are good at some things and not very good at others. All of us have problems, and all of us get illnesses. We all have limitations that keep us from accomplishing most of our dreams. This is the human condition.

Growing Up Is Hard to Do

It is here that we find some of life's hardest lessons and deepest realizations: I am never going to be everything I wanted to be. I am not even going to be able to do everything that I might have done. I simply do not have time to have all the careers I might have wanted, to go all the places I would like to go, to become good at everything I ever wanted to do. I cannot be with all the people I would want to be close to. I have to make choices in life. I pursue some opportunities and not others, but I cannot pursue all the opportunities of life. If I come to a fork in the road, I cannot take both paths. I do one thing, and I don't do all the others I might have done.

When we are young, life does not seem this way. If we are fortunate, people have encouraged us to pursue our dreams. They have seen our potential. They have pointed out our opportunities. When we are young, it seems there is infinite time to do things later. We have thoughts like these: Later, I can go back to college and study something else, or have another career, or learn to fly an airplane, or become a good guitar player, or build a boat and sail around the world.

As life unfolds, most young people feel a sense of progress. Even if they do not like school, they are still likely to go from one grade to the next, from middle school to high school and possibly beyond. Or they graduate from high school and start working as adults. They grow up, learn things, get smarter and stronger and more capable of handling life. By the time most people are young adults, they are nervous but generally optimistic about where they will go and what they will do in life. And if they are lucky, then life keeps progressing. Some people go forward with school or careers, some people fall in love, some people have children and raise them. Many people become more prosperous as they get older. They become "established" in their communities. And even if they are not reaching all of their goals, there is a general sense of progress.

Grief: Where the American Myth Stops

At some point in life, the progress peters out. Eventually, everyone hits the wall. Everyone starts to feel that life might not be an upward cycle of continual progress. At some point, we go as far as we can in our careers. At some point, we realize that we are not going to have time to pursue another career or get another degree. At some point, we find that family relationships are not going to be everything we hoped they would be. At some point, we see our bodies aging and getting weaker rather than getting better and stronger. At some point, we get sick. At some point, we realize that we too are mortal and that we will only get so far in life.

Usually, people hit the wall at some time in midlife, at some point from their late 40s to their mid-60s (Lachman et al. 2015). At this point, bodies and careers and relationships are often topping out, getting near their full potential. Also, at this point in life, most people begin to develop chronic illnesses, such as high blood pressure or arthritis. And at this point, many people experience a deep process of grieving and acceptance. At first, they fight the idea that things cannot always get better, often in classic ways such as having an affair, quitting a job, or buying a new car. But eventually people go from being dissatisfied and restless to being sad and disappointed. They start wondering: Is this all there is? Is this all my life is going to be? If I am "over the hill," does that mean life is all downhill from here? Even if 50 is the new 40, and 40 is the new 30, my life is still going to be limited. I too am human, and I too will experience the human life cycle of growth, maturation, and aging.

In order to go on to deeper levels of growth and maturation, people at this point in life must enter a process of grieving. They tolerate being sad and disappointed, and begin to think about life on a deeper level. They begin to accept themselves as limited and mortal. They come to terms with their flaws and failures and disappointments. They accept that they have illnesses and learn to live with their limitations.

What is so great about all this grieving and acceptance? Grieving what we do not have allows us to accept what we do have and make the most of it. Most of us have not gotten everything we wanted in life, but most of us have gotten more than enough of the good things in life to be happy. The secret of a happy life, if there is one, is to focus on enjoying what we have more than getting what we want. Meanwhile, grieving and acceptance allow us to deal with illness and failure in the best possible way, by getting the help we need and accepting life on its own terms. This does not give us the best possible life, but it gives us the best life that we can possibly have, given all of life's limitations. Going through such a deep process of grief and acceptance gives people a unique kind of wisdom, and a deep knowledge about how to live life. It teaches people the most important things they could ever learn in life.

Mental Illness Is Our Teacher

What does all of this discussion have to do with mental illness? Well, people with mental illness have more of this kind of wisdom than any other group of people I know, and so (in my opinion) people who have come to terms with mental illness have more to teach us about life than any other single group of people I know. Is this because people with mental illness are somehow different from the rest of us? Does mental illness give people uncanny knowledge or psychic powers? Does it teach people something that no one else knows?

Not at all. What people who have accepted mental illness know is what all the rest of us need to know. And the reason people with mental illness know it more deeply and fully than other groups is not because they are a different kind of people. They are the same kind of people, but they have "hit the wall" much earlier in life than almost everyone else, and they have taken a crash course in grief and acceptance in the first part of adulthood. While most people are feeling their oats with energy and optimism as young adults, people with mental illness are getting mental illness. They are hitting the wall.

Unlike most other chronic illnesses, mental illness usually begins when people are in their teens and 20s. Most chronic illnesses begin in middle age or after, but not mental illness. Mental illness usually occurs just as people are entering adulthood (Figure 9–2). There are many exceptions, of course. But the *average age at onset of mental illness is a staggering 14 years*. Fifty percent of all lifetime cases start by age 14, and 75% by age 24 (Kessler et al. 2005). This does not mean that most people with mental illness get diagnosed and treated at age 14. Most people have mental illness for years before they are diagnosed and treated. But looking back, the vast majority of people report that symptoms began in their teens and 20s.

So it turns out that most people develop mental illness in adolescence and young adulthood, times of life that are normally full of optimism and empowerment. While so many young adults are bursting with energy to pursue their dreams, people with mental illness also have to deal with their mental illness. They are hitting the wall and going through one of the greatest transitions in the human lifespan: They are coming to terms with illness, limitation, loss, and failure. We will all have to come to terms with

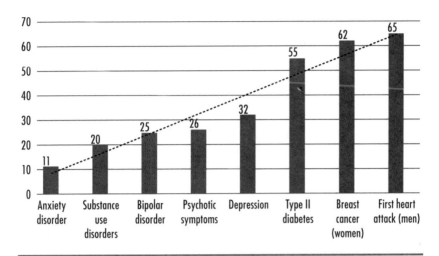

FIGURE 9–2. Average age at onset of common chronic illnesses.

Source. Data from Centers for Disease Control and Prevention 2017; Go et al. 2013; Howlader et al. 2020; Kessler et al. 2005; McGrath et al. 2016; Paus et al. 2008.

these someday, but most who develop mental illness must face these experiences decades before the rest of us.

The process of grief and acceptance is painful beyond words. Most people with moderate to severe mental illnesses will not be able to do everything in life they would have done without those illnesses. Many have dreams that are taken away before they have a chance to pursue them. Mental illness is a bitter pill to swallow, more bitter than any medication. People with mental illness do not choose to have mental illness. But they must face the fact that they will have a life they did not choose, one very different from what they dreamed it could be. They must come to terms with the limitations of life and make a life within those limitations, humbly accepting their fate and their need for help. People dealing with this level of illness must surrender so much of what most people want and expect out of life. What do they get in return for all their pain? The deepest kind of wisdom that life has to offer.

Recovery: Building a Life

Some people never make it to the other side of this transition. Like war, mental illness can cut down people in the prime of life. Many people die before they get a chance to adjust to these harsh realities of life. Some people have so much willpower that they never go through a process of grief and acceptance. They go through life fighting the existence of the illness and refusing treatment, often dying of addiction or schizophrenia or mood disorder. But those who survive and emerge from such a process are like people trying to rebuild a war-torn country. The war is over, but the land is devastated, and rebuilding is a long, bittersweet process. Often, people are starting from scratch, just trying to survive in primitive conditions. Stabilizing from severe mental illness is no easier. It is a daunting process. And yet, sooner or later, rebuilding can begin.

People who are in a process of rebuilding life are described as being in recovery (Leamy et al. 2011). Recovery does not mean that the illness has been cured. It does not mean that the illness does not affect life. Recovery means that people are working with, in, and around the limitations of illness to make a good life for themselves. A good life does not mean a life without illness, without suffering, without failure, without disappointment. A good life is one that accepts all of those things, and within them finds meaning, joy, pleasure, purpose, and connection. No one has a perfectly good life, but on the other hand, no one has to be perfect to have a good life. Instead, people must accept the bad in life while seeking out and dwelling on the good. At the end of twelve-step meetings such as Alcoholic Anonymous, countless groups remind themselves of this truth by joining hands and saying the serenity prayer: "Grant me the serenity to accept the things I cannot change, the courage to change the things I can, and the wisdom to know the difference." This is recovery in a nutshell.

Recovery takes a different path for each person, but the path is always long and winding. Individuals must find the path for themselves, but each will need help from others to walk it. More formally, *recovery* has been defined as "a deeply personal, unique process of changing one's attitudes, values, feelings, goals, skills, and/or roles. It is a way of living a satisfying, hopeful, and contributing life even with limitations caused by illness. Recovery involves the development of new meaning and purpose in one's life as one grows beyond the catastrophic effects of mental illness" (Anthony 1993, p. 257).

Recovery reminds us that people with mental illness are not passive recipients of medical care. They are not incompetent people whose lives need to be controlled. And they are seeking the same things in life as everyone else, overcoming the same kinds of obstacles. Recovery can never be enforced or even given by someone else. Each person must begin a process of grief, acceptance, and recovery within themselves. Each person must consent to or refuse the process of recovery. But no one can recover in isolation. All of us need help and care to overcome problems and illnesses in life.

What People With Mental Illness Can Teach Us

What do people in recovery have to teach us? Most things worth knowing about life, I think. But there is one particular truth gained from recovery that makes me exceedingly grateful: The truth of how to know the measure of a person. What makes a person a success? What makes a good person? Whom should we admire? What standard should we use?

People in recovery know the answers to these questions about the measure of a person. Or rather, they have discarded all the wrong answers. People in recovery know that we as humans cannot measure ourselves by things outside our control. We cannot become arrogant or despairing because of what happens to us in life. We cannot judge ourselves or evaluate ourselves by things we did not choose in life. And strangely enough, the things we cannot choose turn out to have the greatest effects on what we are and what we accomplish in life.

After all, we do not choose our parents. Therefore, we do not choose our genetics either. So we do not get to choose our innate talents or our risk for diseases. We do not choose the basics of our physical appearance. We do not choose our temperament, our level of intelligence, our artistic talent, our athletic talent, or our social abilities. And we do not choose the opportunities that would let us develop our talents and abilities. We do not get to choose the way we grow up. We do not choose our family environment, our culture, our schools, our nutrition, our geography, or our social class. We do not choose our time in history or big events (such as wars or global pandemics) that can determine our fates. We do not create any of the opportunities that come up in life, though we may make our choices in response. Some of us have never had good educational opportunities or good career opportunities or good economic opportunities. And most of all, none of us get to choose our illnesses or our problems in life. If we did, we would probably choose a very different list.

Therefore, the true measure of a person is none of these things. The things we usually associate with success are beauty, wealth, social status, intelligence, power, and charm. These are all nice things to have, but none of them tell us what kind of a person has them. The measure of a person is how that person responds to what they are given in life. Each person is given a "hand of cards" to play in life; the cards include genetics, upbringing, opportunities, and all the rest. The measure of a person is how they are able to accept and play that hand, not how much they win in the game. The true measure of a person is found in how they meet the ups and downs of life, the disappointments and failures, the successes and serendipities that come their way.

What makes a person good? The courage to face painful truths. The determination to keep going even when things look hopeless. The honesty to admit problems. The wisdom to stop blaming others for one's own problems. The humility to seek help outside of oneself. The strength to learn from devastating experiences. The grace to accept one's fate, even when the deck is stacked against the person. People who are recovering from mental illness are not closer to perfect than anyone else. But if they are to survive and rebuild, they have to learn these virtues along the way.

People in recovery understand that personal dignity comes from facing themselves as they are, not from getting status and respect from others. People in recovery understand that living a good life has little to do with success in the conventional sense. People in recovery understand that there is no shame in having problems, no shame in needing help, and no shame in accepting their own limitations. In fact, doing those things makes people truly real, truly good, and truly helpful to others. Because the only way that we as people can truly be of help to others is to work on ourselves, and to admit and address our problems, so that we can be in a position to offer some of what we have learned to others.

Every day, as a practicing psychiatrist, I see people whose lives have been disrupted by mental illness. These people will never be the same, and they will never have exactly the life they would have chosen. But every day, I see these people meet their fate with dignity, nobility, humility, and bravery. Every day, I see such people exercising heroic levels of endurance, grit, and tenacity. Every day, I marvel that they have survived, and that they keep going. Every day, I see them rebuilding their relationships, living situations, careers, and life goals. Every day, I am inspired to emulate them as I face my own trials and adversities. And every day, I notice the ways, large and small, that they make the world around them a better place.

All of this may sound dramatic, but I am speaking literally, not literarily. People who face mental illness and fight their way to recovery have everything the rest of us should admire, and everything we should want to know about life. Maybe it is time to look more deeply at what they have found, time to get past our knee-jerk judgments of those in this situation. Maybe it is time to stop assuming, stop dismissing, and stop advising. Maybe it is time to question our old assumptions about mental illness and the people who deal with it. And maybe it is time for the rest of "us" to start listening to "them."

Advice for Advocacy

- The purpose of this aspect of advocacy is to recognize patients as central and active characters in the drama of illness, treatment, and recovery. By showing that 1) the human experience of illness and limitation is universal, and 2) recovery expresses the highest levels of meaning and human flourishing, you can help the public transition from "those people" to "us people."

- This aspect of advocacy shifts the focus from the pathology and limitation of illness to the active coping and resilience of those who face illness and engage in treatment. Thus, in your advocacy, shift the focus from the deficits to strengths.

- Attempt to walk the delicate line between acknowledging the unique experiences of those who face mental illness (on one hand) and articulating that everyone in life faces similar challenges (on the other).

- Some patients and family members are understandably sensitive to terminology. Avoid calling a group of people "schizophrenics" or "the mentally ill," which could imply that the disorder defines the person, or that we are dealing with a different order of person—something very different than "people who have schizophrenia" or "those who deal with mental illness."

- Remember, you are not lecturing others on recovery. Acknowledge and appreciate those brave enough to walk this difficult path.

- Consider your own patients and what you have learned from those in recovery. Ask yourself how you would fare in their life circumstances, and look for things to admire about the ways they have faced their life challenges.

- In order to deeply appreciate the achievements of those in recovery, you must come to terms with your own personal limitations, problems, and illnesses. You will need to appreciate both your limitations and ways you have learned to live well in their presence.

- In the same way, if you cannot personally give up ideas of human perfectibility and unlimited achievement, then you will implicitly characterize the limitations of illness as shameful inadequacies.

References

Alcoholics Anonymous: Alcoholics Anonymous: The Big Book, 4th Edition. New York, AA World Services, 2001

Anthony WA: Recovery from mental illness: the guiding vision of the mental health service system in the 1990s. Psychosocial Rehabilitation Journal 16(4):11–23, 1993

Centers for Disease Control and Prevention: National Diabetes Statistics Report, 2017. Atlanta, GA, Centers for Disease Control and Prevention, U.S. Dept of Health and Human Services, 2017

Go AS, Mozaffarian D, Roger VL, et al: Heart disease and stroke statistics—2013 update: a report from the American Heart Association. Circulation 127:e6–e245, 2013

Howlader N, Noone AM, Krapcho M, et al (eds): SEER Cancer Statistics Review (CSR) 1975–2016. National Cancer Institute, April 9, 2020. Available at: https://seer.cancer.gov/csr/1975_2016/. Accessed August 4, 2020.

Kessler RC, Berglund P, Demler O, et al: Lifetime prevalence and age-of-onset distributions of DSM-IV disorders in the National Comorbidity Survey Replication. Arch Gen Psychiatry 62(6):593–602, 2005

Lachman ME, Teshale S, Agrigoroaei S: Midlife as a pivotal period in the life course: balancing growth and decline at the crossroads of youth and old age. Int J Behav Dev 39(1):20–31, 2015

Leamy M, Bird V, Le Boutillier C, et al: Conceptual framework for personal recovery in mental health: systematic review and narrative synthesis. Br J Psychiatry 199(6):445–452, 2011

McGrath JJ, Saha S, Al-Hamzawi AO, et al: Age of onset and lifetime projected risk of psychotic experiences: cross-national data from the World Mental Health Survey. Schizophr Bull 42(4):933–941, 2016

Paus T, Keshavan M, Giedd JN: Why do many psychiatric disorders emerge during adolescence? Nat Rev Neurosci 9(12):947–957, 2008

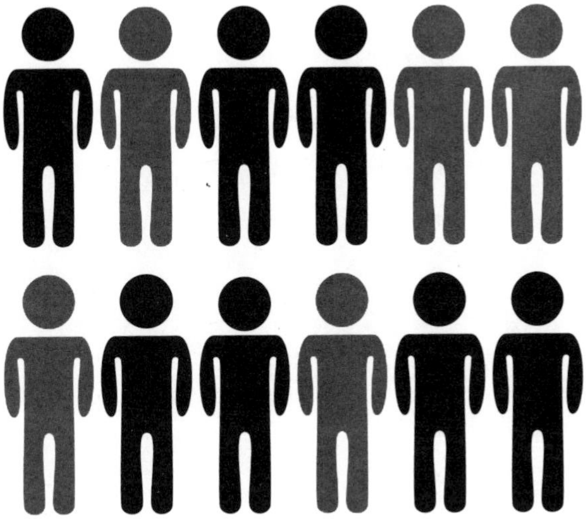

10

Afterword:
A Vision of
Unity

What is the endpoint of advocacy? The endpoint is the universal and matter-of-fact recognition that mental illness is a common and treatable form of medical illness. This sounds quite modest, but it turns out that the truth about mental illness is far more difficult to accept and integrate than its simplicity implies. Shame, stigma, bias, misunderstanding, minimization, and denial remain to this day. So the full intellectual, emotional, and social integration of these truths will be a substantial accomplishment, one that will put an end to stigma and the second-class treatment of mental health care.

The way toward this endpoint is defined by openness and honesty: As a culture we cannot integrate the truth about mental illness without admitting that "we," individually and socially, are the ones dealing with mental illness. And as professionals, we cannot effectively lead the way without admitting that we too are part of that "us." The existence of a "them" (the "mentally ill") who are separate from "us" (the "normals" and the helpers) indicates that "we" are still projecting our sense of brokenness and vulnerability onto "them" rather than accepting it. Such a habit shows that bias and stigma still exist, and will exist until we lose this sense of fundamental difference from those with illness. When we all come to share a sense of both strength and weakness, and when we can take various social and medical roles without losing this sense, we will know that a new era has come. When there is no more "them" in regard to mental health, we will know we have arrived. And then the real work can go forward.

A Common Way Forward

The evidence is overwhelming.

- Mental illness is common: It affects us all.
- Mental illness is real: It is as real as any other medical illness.
- Mental illness is serious: It is as deadly and disabling as any type of medical illness.
- Mental illness is nobody's fault: No one should be blamed for it.
- Mental illness is treatable: It is as treatable as other chronic illnesses.

These truths are not self-evident; they cut against what used to be common sense. But they are scientifically grounded. They are scientifically justified, justified beyond a reasonable doubt. The evidence is overwhelming. The evidence is so great that no one could read and evaluate all of the studies in one lifetime. And findings from new, more advanced studies are reported every day.

We now know a vast amount about mental illness. Over a century ago, psychiatrist Carl Jung called psychology "a fortuitous conglomeration of unscientific opinions" (Jung 1921/1976, p. 987). There have always been a lot of people with a lot to say about mental illness and the mind. But what we know now is no mere conglomeration of opinions. We now have a scientific foundation for understanding mental health and mental illness. That foundation is based on so many studies over so many years that it is not going to be contradicted or undermined. Instead, we will slowly, painstakingly upgrade and build on that foundation.

Still, we do not know everything about mental illness. We do not know most of the things we really need to know about it. I am certain that we *don't* know more about mental illness than we *do* know. But this is not discouraging. We are studying the most complex object in the physical universe. We began by talking about the complexity of the human brain, and we will end with it as well. If there is a true final frontier in the universe, it is a human being, and the very hub of what it takes to be human is the human brain. Researchers will be working to understand the human brain and mental illness for many decades to come, longer than any of us will be alive.

So this is not the end of the story, the end of the maze that takes us to an understanding of mental illness. We are not at the end, but we are not at the beginning either. In my opinion, we are at the end of the beginning. We are now done with false starts, with theories based on raw observations and opinions, with dogmatic belief in one system over another, and with sterile debates over mind vs. body, heredity vs. environment, medication vs. psychotherapy. We have a foundation, a true scientific basis to move forward. We are entering the middle phase of this centuries-long quest—the quest of human beings to understand the human condition, to understand the mind, and to understand mental illness.

We will never go back to the stigma of the past. And there is no need to return to debates about the "myth of mental illness" or "toxic psychiatry." Instead, the questions and disagreements that remain will simply spur on more research and scientific advancement. But advancement will be slower and more complicated in mental illness than in any other field of scientific endeavor, because if we want to understand mental illness, we have to understand the human mind, the human brain, human society, and the human spirit. We have to understand the deepest mysteries of who and what we are.

Most importantly, we now have a way of going forward together. We still need debate and disagreement. We need people to challenge traditional ideas and practices among mental health professionals, to question the way we do things, and to demand a better way forward. But we do not have to go back to square one, start over, or disagree about the fundamentals of what we are doing. What we are doing is working together to address the needs of those with mental illness and their families. And the way we are doing that is on the basis of medical, psychological, and social research to develop medical, psychological, and social treatments to treat medical, psychological, and social problems. We now know the basics of what we are treating, and how we are going to go about improving our understanding and treatments. We are now all in the position to be on the same side: the side of those who happen to be dealing with mental illness.

All of this is excellent news. For the first time in human history, the nature of mental illness is beyond reasonable debate. Mental illness is medical illness affecting the whole person, and mental health treatment is medical, psychological, and social treatment that addresses the whole person. No one is to blame for mental illness. No one needs to be ashamed. No one needs to be stigmatized. We are now on the threshold of something that seemed like a pipe dream 50 years ago: treating mental illness like any other kind of medical illness, treating people with mental illness like people with any other kind of medical illness, and working together to address this problem like any other medical and social problem.

All Together Now

Sigmund Freud may have been sexually abused as a child. He most certainly had panic attacks and phobias as an adult (Jones 1961). He was the most famous psychiatrist in history. The second most famous was his understudy, Carl Jung. Jung suffered from something very close to psychotic depression in 1912, shortly after his breakup with Sigmund Freud (Jung 1963). He had a long family history of extremely eccentric, possibly psychotic ancestors (Bair 2004). William James, America's most famous psychologist, had suicidal depression and panic (McDermott 1967/1977). John Watson, a founder of behaviorist psychology, was distant and estranged from his children. One of his daughters and two of his sons attempted suicide. A granddaughter, the actress Mariette Hartley, went on to become an advocate for mental health as honorary director of the American Foundation for Suicide Prevention (Hartley and Commire 1990). What about mental health professionals today? Kay Redfield Jamison, one of the leading experts on bipolar disorder, has written movingly about her own bipolar disorder (Jamison 1995). And Marsha Linehan, the psychologist behind the best proven treatment for borderline personality disorder, has publicly discussed her own borderline personality disorder (Linehan 2020).

And though it is slightly beside the point, one of my favorite stories along these lines is about two other psychiatrists, Karl and William Menninger. Karl wrote best-selling books about mental health, and William appeared on the October 25, 1948, cover of *Time Magazine*. They were the most respected and powerful American psychiatrists of the post–World War II era, and together they ran the Menninger Clinic. Yet the story is told that their mother would occasionally visit them at work. There they would be, deciding the fate of American psychiatry. Yet when the call came in that Mother was approaching, they would snuff out their cigarettes, hide the ashtrays, and open up the office windows—Mother, it seems, did not know they smoked, and they were terrified she would find out (Friedman 1990)!

What is my point? My point is that we do not need to try and separate those with mental illness from doctors, psychotherapists, and researchers. Nor do we need to distinguish them from family members and advocates. We are all in this together. The dividing lines between doctors, therapists, patients, family members, researchers, advocates, and members of the general public are illusory. Most us will fill more than one of these roles in the course of our lifetime. People with mental illness *are* doctors, family members, researchers, and advocates, just as often as are people without mental illness. People with mental illness *are* the general public. People with mental illness are not "those people," they are "us people," because there is no meaningful social group that does not contain people with mental illness. And so we cannot separate people with mental illness from doctors, family members, and the rest. Whether or not we as individuals have had mental illness, we all care about people with mental illness personally, and so we all care about mental illness in a personal way. It is a problem for all of us, and addressing this problem is important to all of us. Finding solutions to that problem will benefit all of us personally.

Sometimes when thinking about such things, I recall a scene from the 1960 movie *Spartacus. Spartacus* is loosely based on the true story of the greatest slave revolt in the Roman Empire, led by a gladiator named Spartacus. Spartacus and his fellow slaves freed themselves and defeated several Roman armies before Spartacus was captured along with many other rebel soldiers. In the movie, the Romans are not sure which prisoner is Spartacus; naturally, there are no photographs or facial recognition software programs to help them out. Finally, the Romans prepare to kill everyone unless Spartacus comes forward. So Spartacus (played by Kirk Douglas) slowly pulls himself to his feet, ready to admit in defeat that he is Spartacus. But just as he opens his mouth, someone else jumps up and loudly claims to be Spartacus. Spartacus just stares at him, but meanwhile someone else has jumped up and announced that he too is Spartacus. Another slave does the same, and another, until finally all the prisoners are on their feet, shouting and insisting that all of them are Spartacus. The Romans are dumbfounded.

Someday, I feel certain, this is going to happen in regard to mental illness. Maybe it has already started to happen, because in such a vast culture it is hard to tell. In all sorts of rooms, all sorts of times and places, one person is going to stand up and say, "I am affected by mental illness. I have it; my child has it; my best friend has it." But before the first person has stopped speaking, the next will jump up and say, "I am affected by mental illness." And another will say so, and another, until finally a wave of recognition will sweep over the room: We are all affected—all of us. And a balance will tip, and everyone in the room, everyone in the community, and indeed everyone in the country is going to realize that mental illness is no longer about "those people." It is not "those people" who have to deal with mental illness, and it is not "those people" who need our help. It is "us" and it is all people. When enough brave people speak up (as so many already have), then a moment will come when people look around and see that they are no longer in the minority. They no longer have to be afraid that "someone will know" or "they wouldn't understand." They will have to understand, because "they" are all affected, every bit as much as the rest of us. And when that moment comes, when that balance tips, it is never going back. The reality of mental illness is based on truth, on something real that can never be unseen once it has been seen. And once we have all seen it, as a society, a culture, a nation, and a world, it will be too real and obvious for words, much less debate. We will finally realize that mental illness is part of being human, of having a body and a brain, and of getting sick. Mental illness is simply part of the human condition, a condition common to us all. And then, at last, we will go forward together.

References

Bair D: Jung: A Biography. Boston, MA, Back Bay Books, 2004
Friedman LJ: Menninger: The Family and the Clinic. New York, Knopf, 1990
Hartley M, Commire A: Breaking the Silence. New York, Putnam, 1990
Jamison KR: An Unquiet Mind: A Memoir of Moods and Madness. New York, Knopf, 1995
Jones E: The Life and Work of Sigmund Freud. Edited and abridged by Trilling L, Marcus S. New York, Basic Books, 1961
Jung CG: Psychological Types (1921). Princeton, NJ, Princeton University Press, 1976
Jung CG: Memories, Dreams, Reflections. New York, Vintage, 1963
Linehan MM: Building a Life Worth Living: A Memoir. New York, Random House, 2020
McDermott JJ: The Writings of William James: A Comprehensive Edition (1967). Chicago, IL, University of Chicago Press, 1977

Index

Page numbers printed in **boldface** type refer to tables or figures.